MW00595714

THE BIG BLACK BOOK OF
sex
POSITIONS

Take Your Sex Life From
Boring To Mind-Blowing
in a Few More Than 69 Moves

Jennifer Baritchi and Rob Alex, PhD

Images by
Andrew Poplavsky

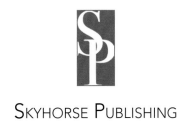

SKYHORSE PUBLISHING

Copyright © 2019 by Jennifer Baritchi and Rob Alex, PhD

All rights reserved. No part of this book may be reproduced in any manner without the express written consent of the publisher, except in the case of brief excerpts in critical reviews or articles. All inquiries should be addressed to Skyhorse Publishing, 307 West 36th Street, 11th Floor, New York, NY 10018.

Skyhorse Publishing books may be purchased in bulk at special discounts for sales promotion, corporate gifts, fund-raising, or educational purposes. Special editions can also be created to specifications. For details, contact the Special Sales Department, Skyhorse Publishing, 307 West 36th Street, 11th Floor, New York, NY 10018 or info@skyhorsepublishing.com.

Skyhorse® and Skyhorse Publishing® are registered trademarks of Skyhorse Publishing, Inc.®, a Delaware corporation.

Visit our website at www.skyhorsepublishing.com.

10 9 8 7 6 5 4 3

Images by Andrew Poplavsky

Library of Congress Cataloging-in-Publication Data is available on file.

Cover design by Mona Lin

ISBN: 978-1-5107-4006-8
EISBN: 978-1-5107-4007-5

Printed in China

THE BIG BLACK BOOK OF

sex

POSITIONS

CONTENTS

INTRODUCTION

IN THE BEGINNING THERE WAS SEX, BASIC AND PRIMAL IN ITS EARLY STAGES, OR SO WE THINK. . . . Perhaps modern society is simply unaware of the depth of sexual understanding our ancestors truly possessed. Maybe modern society is actually relearning the sexual secrets that have been lost over the years. We can look back to the Kama Sutra and see that thousands of years ago, the various sexual positions were given extreme importance. There are even ancient texts that suggest certain positions and angles of penetration can improve your health, and even fight disease—providing more than just physical pleasure. However, intense physical pleasure is an excellent place to start.

The basic missionary position gets the job done, and is quite enjoyable, but year after year of the same sexual position can become boring and less stimulating. It's like eating the same amazing chocolate cake for dessert every night. After a while, it starts to taste bland and we lose our desire for that chocolate cake. So when we try another dessert like strawberry shortcake, the strawberries seem to explode with flavor. Why should sex be any different?

As you explore the more than one hundred different sex positions in this book, you'll notice that each position creates a new and unique sensation in your body and mind, resulting in different and exciting lovemaking experiences that keep the passion alive and your sex life thriving.

All of your senses will be heightened as you explore many new sexual positions. Your sense of touch takes center stage when trying new and different positions. You may find one magic position that allows her to finally experience a vaginal or G-spot orgasm, and another position that allows him to last a little longer while still enjoying full penetration. Visual pleasure and stimulation are also amplified as you are able to enjoy your partner from new angles and perspectives. As you venture away from the standard missionary position, you will be able to hear your partner in all their pleasure in new and exciting ways. As we move into oral sex and other positions that will allow you to kiss and lick previously unexplored areas of your partner's body, your taste buds will dance with joy. And lastly, there is nothing more erotic than the smell of pure raw sex as you and your partner emit your own delicious scent of orgasmic bliss.

Aren't you starting to see how powerful this book is going to be in igniting your sex life and keeping the passion alive?

One of the greatest pleasures for you and your partner will be the fun and adventure you experience together as you try to figure out exactly how to get into each position, and what each new position does or does not do for you. Don't be afraid to have fun on this journey! There will be laughter and giggles coming from your bedroom, as we know for a fact that there will be times that you fall over or end up looking like a pretzel as you work through the positions this book. That's OK—sex is supposed to be fun. Don't ever forget that!

At the end of each chapter, you'll find a "Sexy Challenge" to expand and further enhance the enjoyment of your sexual experiences. Each Sexy Challenge teaches you to look at sex not only as a biological act, but as an emotional and spiritual experience. So open your mind and your body to the possibilities of something more . . . something exciting and truly orgasmic.

We hope this book and all of the positions and adventures inside add much more passion and fun to your sex life. And, in addition, it will create something special and magical for each and every one of you. Take the risk, and at least try each and every one of these positions. It will create a deeper sexual connection with your lover, as well as a more intimate, stronger love for one another.

SPECIAL NOTE

We want to take just a moment to address an obvious concern that some of you will have about this book. All of the positions in this book portray a male–female heterosexual couple, where the male partner is generally the dominant partner. We chose this approach because it appeals to the largest group of people, but that is in no way the only group who can get extreme enjoyment from this book.

All of the positions can be modified to work with same sex partners and even more than one partner. This is where sex really gets fun and interesting. Our personal motto is to try everything at least twice, because the first time learning a new skill is always awkward. Normally, after the third try, you'll really know if you love it or hate it.

- If you're generally dominant, let your partner take control.

- If you've never tried anal sex, try it and you'll know for sure whether or not you enjoy it.

- Switch roles to get in touch with your previously unexplored masculine or feminine side.

- Try as many different toys and props as you can get your hands on.

Our personal challenge to you is to have fun with your partner or partners, and try each of these positions from every different angle and role. You will be surprised how much more enjoyable sex will be when you can get out of your personal comfort zone and truly open up to new sexual experiences with your partner.

Peace, Love, and Joy,

Jennifer Baritchi and Rob Alex, PhD

CHAPTER 1: FOREPLAY DONE RIGHT

WHAT IS FOREPLAY?

By definition, foreplay is any sexual activity that precedes intercourse, but this is setting you up for failure. This definition sets you up for a very monotonous and predictable sex life. Foreplay is about much more than just the actions that immediately preceded the penis entering the vagina. Here's another approach—one that's guaranteed to keep sex fun and exciting, even if you've been married for thirty years.

> New definition of foreplay: Any sexual play that takes sex from boring to mind blowing. It occurs before, during, and after sexual intercourse.

Sex is supposed to be fun, but far too many people take sexual play way too seriously. It's time to get out of the mindset that foreplay is just a motion we go through before we have sex. Foreplay is so many things! It is flirting, teasing, sucking, groping, fondling, squeezing, licking, kissing. The list goes on and on. Foreplay is something that happens all day long. It happens during sex, and it happens after sex. Foreplay is an attitude and a personality that should be living and breathing inside all of us. It's what makes sex really fun and exciting.

ALL-DAY FOREPLAY

If you think that foreplay is just a warm-up exercise to sex, you are missing out on a lot of amazing pleasure. Get your mind out of robotic human mode, and start understanding that pleasure is an energy that doesn't have a beginning and ending point. Foreplay is a continuous activity. It starts when we wake up, and ends when we go to sleep, as we are sharing this sexual energy exchange all day long. From the first kiss in the morning, to the lingering hugs as we fall asleep. Every action and feeling you direct towards your lover is foreplay, and what you do at 9 a.m. in the morning can have a huge impact on if and how you enjoy sex in the evening.

You see, real foreplay doesn't just happen in the minutes before you start having sexual intercourse. Every kiss, every sexy look, every email or text, every time you brush up against your partner is foreplay. But it doesn't stop there. Foreplay continues while you are having sex and long after. You can call this "after play" if it makes easier to grasp the concept, but immediately after sex, you begin foreplay for the next time you're together. There is no stopping or starting point. Truly amazing sex is a continuous ebb and flow of energy. All the actions you take now will have a direct impact on the next time, and the next.

So, if you roll over and just fall asleep immediately after sex, you're missing a valuable opportunity to set the tone for your next sexual encounter. Understanding that you are ALWAYS having foreplay with your partner is something that will keep your relationship happy and healthy, and ensure that your sex life stays fresh and exciting.

Think about all the amazing memories you have as a couple. Every time you laugh together, foreplay. Every time you hug, foreplay. Every time you fight, foreplay. In some sense, every interaction you have with a lover is foreplay. Think about it. If you piss your partner off, you are most likely not having sex tonight, unless it's makeup sex. But if you do something special for your partner, your chances of getting laid go way up!

Now that you understand that everything you do is foreplay, it's time to start thinking about every action you take while you're with them. That is, if you enjoy having hot, steamy sex with your partner.

If you take this approach to foreplay, you will see amazing benefits to your relationship and your sex life. Getting turned on is so much easier, because you've been thinking about and wanting your partner for hours or days. It will be easier to make your partner wet or give them an erection. Every action and energy transfer, from the last time you had sex to the present, have a direct and very powerful impact.

THE WARM UP

Remember: If you want to have amazing sex all the time, the foreplay never stops. It may sound like a lot of work, but the rewards are well worth it. Seriously, who wouldn't want amazing sex with their partner? So stop being lazy and put some effort into it!

Now that you understand how important all your actions are leading up to the time when you're ready to have sexual intercourse—you know "Tab A into Slot B;" now we can focus more on the specific actions of foreplay as a sexual warm up.

To get the body physically ready for sex we need to increase blood flow to all of the sexual areas—not only the genitals, but all of the other erogenous zones on your partner's body. Think of the places on your partner's body that get them really aroused.

THE MOST COMMON EROGENOUS ZONES FOR WOMEN

- Ankles and feet
- Breast and nipples
- Clitoris, the whole organ and not just the tip
- Ears and the nape of her neck
- Hands and wrists
- Inner thighs, especially up high
- Inside of the arm near the elbow and under arm
- Mouth and lips
- Stomach, especially the lower abdomen

THE MOST COMMON EROGENOUS ZONES FOR MEN

- His butt cheeks. It's not fair that the girls get all the attention.

- Ears and the nape of his neck

- Mouth and lips

- Nipples

- Penis and scrotum

- Prostate, both inside and outside the anus

- Lower abdomen

Be adventurous and let go of any prudish baggage that you may have been taught as a child. Sex is supposed to be fun!

Seek out all ways that get blood flowing in your partner's body to these erogenous zones. While in the warm-up mode, feel free to use any and all methods at your disposal including your hands, mouth, tongue, fingers, nose, and even your toes. Any part of your body can be used for foreplay. And don't forget toys. Anything that stimulates your partner and turns them on is fair game. And don't forget that you can also stimulate yourself at the same time.

FUCKING PLAY

After the Warm Up, you can move into foreplay during actual sex! Let's just call this Fucking Play. If you're just having sex by moving the penis in and out of the vagina, you are missing out on amazing "play" during this time.

Any action you take at this point is doubled on the intensity scale. Sucking on your partner's nipples, sticking a finger in their anus, and talking dirty to them, all score bonus points while you are actually making love to them.

During Fucking Play, you can get away with something you might not have been able to during the Warm Up. You can smack that ass a little harder, or talk a little dirtier to them. All the walls seem to come down a little bit in the throes of passion.

ORGASM PLAY

The next form of play is Orgasm Play. This is when your partner is actually in the middle of orgasming. This can be the hardest form of play because, as your partner is having an orgasm, they will fight the added pleasure of additional play. The intense feeling just gets to be too much, and they have to push you away at some point.

While you want to keep the pleasure flowing, the body of your partner at some point says, "too much pleasure overload" and it reacts by stopping you. This is the point that most people think all play stops, and they are so wrong. Those that actually stop here are making a huge mistake. The After Play can be amazing and a true way to connect in a deeper manner with our partner, not to mention providing the added benefit of a second or third orgasm!

AFTER PLAY

After your partner has their orgasm or several orgasms, many people think sexual activity is over. This is actually when "after play" begins. After Play is not designed to get your partner aroused again; however sometimes that does actually happen. After Play is about helping your partner's body come back from sexual bliss to its normal position. Instead of going from the shock to the body of having an orgasm to just everything stopping, the After Play is designed to help your partner gradually come back from the most amazing place. You have to understand that an orgasm is a journey to the farthest reaches of the universe and back again in just a few seconds. If you are smart and caring, you have to help your partner return from this blissful place.

After Play is very similar to foreplay, except in reverse. We are taking our partner's genital arousal back to the relaxed state. After Play is about connection and love. After play can be as simple as cleaning up your partner with a towel, or wiping all the juices away in a gentle and loving fashion. It can also be about touching each other, connecting, and allowing our bodies to return to a place of normality. At this point the penis doesn't have to be erect, and the pussy doesn't have to be wet, and yet there is still an amazing sexual exchange between lovers. This sexual exchange is more of a spiritual experience than a physical one, yet both have this blissful feeling that leaves you in awe.

SETTING THE MOOD IN FIVE EASY STEPS

Getting yourself, as well as your partner, in the mood is an art in its own right. First of all, you might know what would work for you, but we are not only concerned with 'your' mood. You have another person to consider, and while you might have very specific things that get you in the mood, those might not work as well for your partner. So we have a balancing act that we have to deal with. How much of what we want and desire do we put into, and combine with, what we know our partner might like and enjoy? The sad part is there is no perfect formula, but that is also good, because each attempt at setting the mood can be unique and exciting each and every time.

So often when we hear the term "Setting the Mood," we associate it with just the act of sex. Well there are all kinds of things you can set the mood for, and yes, sex is one of those. You can also set the mood for romance, for a surprise, or even some big news, like promotions at work or winning a vacation; so you first have to know exactly what your setting the mood for. With that, we have tried to break it down to allow you the ability to set the mood for any and every occasion with five simple steps. So, these steps are vague and open to all types of moods you are trying to create.

An important part of anything you do is to put your unique stamp on it. So don't try to be someone you're not. If you're a happy-go-lucky person, don't try to be downright serious. If you're not a literary ace, then you might not want to express things with poetry. Believe me, those poems that start with "There once was a man from Nantucket" usually don't set the right mood. Allow your personality to come through when you're setting the mood, but always look for something different new and/or exciting to throw off your partner a little, so they know you are growing and improving as a lover. We want them to be a little on their toes and not expect the same old thing over and over again.

The big thing to remember is that it isn't easy to set a specific mood. Your partner might not react to things you set in place the way you would expect them to, so you can't get into the mindset of thinking you know what reactions your partner will have to any given situation. Expecting a specific reaction will just stall any mood you are desiring to create. The best mood setters are quick to react and change things up, hopefully bringing the mood back where you intended it to go. Know that sometimes, however, the best mood-setting techniques will not work. Sometimes they will go a completely different direction, or something will happen to derail the mood completely. Those things might be a sick child, a bad day at work, or you could have done something to really piss off your partner earlier in the day, so that nothing you do will change that mood. Plus, there are endless outside forces that can affect the mood setting. However, when you achieve your goal of setting a specific mood, especially for sex, all will seem right in the world.

Okay, enough gibber-gabber, it is time to get to work with our five easy steps to setting the mood. Once you get this process down, you can really start to add and adjust things to make each experience a sensational work of art.

STEP #1: GET EXCITED ABOUT SETTING THE MOOD—You will never set the correct mood with half-assed attempts. You should actually get more and more excited about it as the process goes along. I suggest starting out by visualizing the end result and working backwards. For example, if your goal is to have some amazing and freaky sex, then imagine that you are both in bed exhausted and very satisfied, and then start working your way backwards. Thinking about what got you into bed, and then what happened before that, and so on and so forth, until you get a picture of what you hope to accomplish. This can be a meditation of sorts or maybe even a visualization of what you want to happen. I base this off the first rule of Huna that states, "The World is What You Think It is."

Now allow your mind, body, and spirit to get excited about what you are going to plan, or attempt to plan out. There is an amazing energy that comes out when you get excited. This energy will help you make the most out of setting the mood. Plus, when you're excited about what you are doing, that energy will spill over into your partner and they will ride that wave as well. Put simply, the more excited you are about setting the mood, the better it usually turns out. The more excited you are about this, the more effort you will put into it, and that will show greatly to your partner.

STEP #2: A BASIC PLAN—Once you are excited about the mood you want to be setting, the next step is to create a basic plan. By that I mean you need to have an outline of specific things you want to do to set the mood. You need to avoid making it too specific, to the point where the entire evening is planned out. Planning out every little detail will lead to your mood setting seeming stale and feeling too staged. You need to have room for spontaneity, and allow the evening to evolve in the most amazing ways. If you try to follow a rigid schedule, anything can throw you off your game, so you have to be open to the flow of the evening.

My suggestion is making a few bullet points of things you might want to do. Plan out about four to five things you want to use to set the mood, and set them up to be launched when the time is right. One of my favorite things to do is to place flower petals on a ceiling fan and then, when you are your partner are under the fan, turn it on, leaving you both standing in a light rain of flower petals. This type of action can be set up in advance and can happen at any point in the evening, and is especially good if your ceiling fan is over your bed, wink wink. When trying to make your basic plan, avoid trying to stick to a time schedule, so don't incorporate going to the movies or reservations into your plan. Those steps will force your actions and you want to share them only in due time.

Don't try to cram too much into your basic plan because when you try to do too much, it becomes a little overwhelming not only for yourself, but for your partner as well. When too much is planned, your partner doesn't have the time to really enjoy the things you are using to set the mood. Plus, this way you get to save some of your interesting ideas for the next time you are creating your mood-setting plan.

STEP #3: TEASE—Now that your plan is in place, it is time to start the teasing process. Now, by teasing, we don't mean doing it in an obvious fashion. Your teasing should be subtle depending on the mood you are trying to set. Teasing can be as simple as making kisses last a little longer, holding hands when you normally wouldn't, or even touching your partner in a sensual way. You can tease your partner by giving them compliments, and going out of your way to do things for them. Simply doing a chore that your partner usually completes is a great way to get their attention as to what you are up to. Anything that disrupts the flow of a normal day could be considered teasing and leading up to setting the mood you so desire.

Another great way to tease your partner is by leaving them a note in a place they will find it when you are not around. This will let them know you are thinking about them, even when you are not around, and it won't be too much of a tease as to what is to follow later on. You can also send them a text message that doesn't make much sense to get them curious. Something like, "Do we have any whipped cream at home?" These type of text messages will get your partner's mind wondering just exactly what you're up to. A curious mind will be open to all kinds of possibilities. Now, with teasing, you need to avoid giving away too much, like telling them "I have something amazing in store for you tonight." You don't want to give away too much. You just want your partner to be a little curious.

When you master the art of teasing, you will have an amazing benefit in your corner. You will soon know exactly what to say and do to make your partner very interested in what might happen, but you will be able to keep it secret enough that they will have a surprise waiting for them. Teasing leads to another great feature called anticipation, and when you get your partner anticipating something is going to happen, and you can draw it out, you can direct them towards the mood you are looking to set.

STEP #4: TAKE IT SLOW—It is easy to want to rush into everything we have set up at this point. Especially if you have really focused on getting excited yourself. You will be so hopped up on energy that you might want to just get to it. Setting a mood is just like acting, telling a joke, singing a song, etc., where the timing is super important. There are reasons for dramatic pauses and a little silence before the punch line. These are to heighten the sensation of the acting or joke. Think about that when you find yourself rushing through any part of setting the mood. The experiences that are happening during this process are to be savored and not completed as fast as possible.

Trust me when I tell you, the slower you go, the better and more exciting the end results will be. You have to allow time for your partner to enjoy the process.

Sometimes your partner will try to speed things up. For example, if you're setting a sexy mood and you partner starts getting a little more excited than expected, you might have to calm them down just a little so that they don't rush through the process. Believe me, it is hard when that happens not to just abandon all your planning and allow things to progress quicker. However, remember savoring these moments will make them last in time, and build even more anticipation and desire. So, have some self-control and assure your partner you are going to get there, but they need to allow you to slow it down a little and let the anticipation build to an even hotter level.

STEP #5: IN THE END, LET PASSION RUN WILD—Once all is said and done, it is time to let passion take over. Once you have set the mood you have been going for, it is time to let the horses run free. If you're going for a sexy mood, it is time to let the kiss get deep and your hands explore your partner's body. If it's a romantic mood you are going for, then it is time to dig deep and pull out the most soulful kiss you have ever shared with anyone, and it is time to gaze into their eyes. Passion can take many forms at this time, so don't be afraid to laugh act silly or just plain get crazy. No matter how all your plans turned out, if your partner truly loves and cares about you, they will be so appreciative of what you have done, that you are going to get lucky.

In every relationship I have ever been in, I took great pride in trying to make moments special. Now, we can't make every moment special in our relationship, but the ones we do make special are the ones that will be remembered forever. A moment that is remembered forever is one that will always bring a smile to your face, and will always take you back to the mood that was created.

CHAPTER 2: MISSIONARY SEX POSITIONS

MISSIONARY

The "chicken soup" of sex positions, the Missionary is an old favorite enjoyed by many couples. In fact, it's probably the first position you've ever tried and might still be your go-to sex position when you just want to experience something familiar. Both partners enjoy this sex position!

HOW TO DO IT

The missionary position is often also called "man on top," and rightly so. The male partner assumes the dominant position on top of the woman, who is lying on her back. Her legs are spread enough so that her lover can thrust, but they're not raised up or resting on his shoulders. While there, she can thrust some, but the primary work done here is by the man.

WHERE TO DO IT

The sofa, bed, and floor are all great locations for this position, but it can be done anywhere the two of you can lie down comfortably.

PROPS YOU'LL NEED

A pillow under her lower back can help support her hips and tilt her pelvis so that penetration is more comfortable and pleasurable.

DIFFICULTY LEVEL ★☆☆☆☆

HER O-METER ★★★☆☆

While this is a great position for intimacy and connection, it's not the most physically stimulating position. Some of the variations that we'll cover shortly are much better for her stimulation and orgasm potential. Having said that, it's one of the most common positions, so here are a few tips to make it better. She can vary the angle and height of her hips to get better depth and angle of penetration. Another option is moving her hips up and down, back and forth, or even in circles to better stimulate her sensitive areas.

HIS O-METER ★★★★☆

He fares much better in the Missionary position than she does, simply because he can control the speed and depth of penetration, and he is able to orgasm how and when he wants to.

The trick here is to make sure that she is really turned on, so that she wants to devour her partner. If you find that she is just lying there and not responding, then back off and spend a little more time getting her turned on first so that you can both enjoy this position more.

Focus on the intimacy and emotional connection afforded by the missionary position. Leave the lights on and gaze into each other's eyes. Focus on the sensation of each and every thrust. There will be plenty of other opportunities to get raw and primal. This type of intimacy is totally hot and allows both partners to fully connect emotionally, which is not always so easy to do!

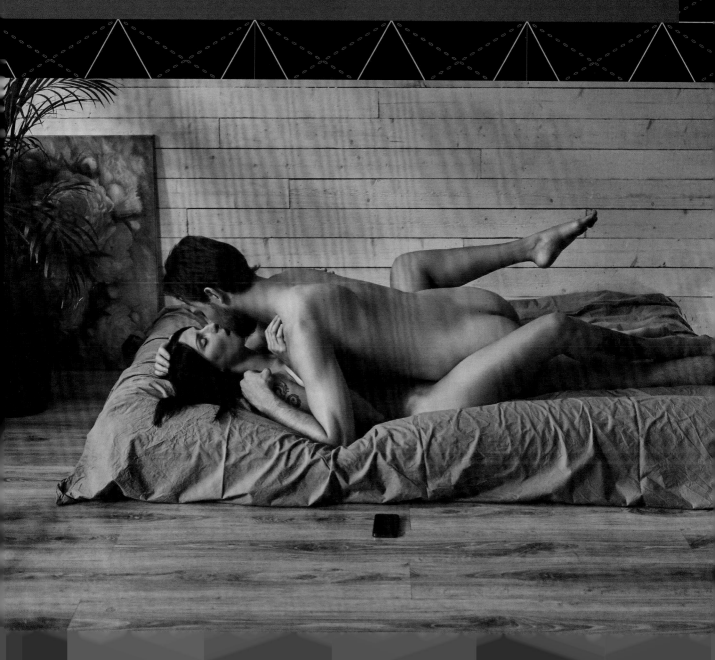

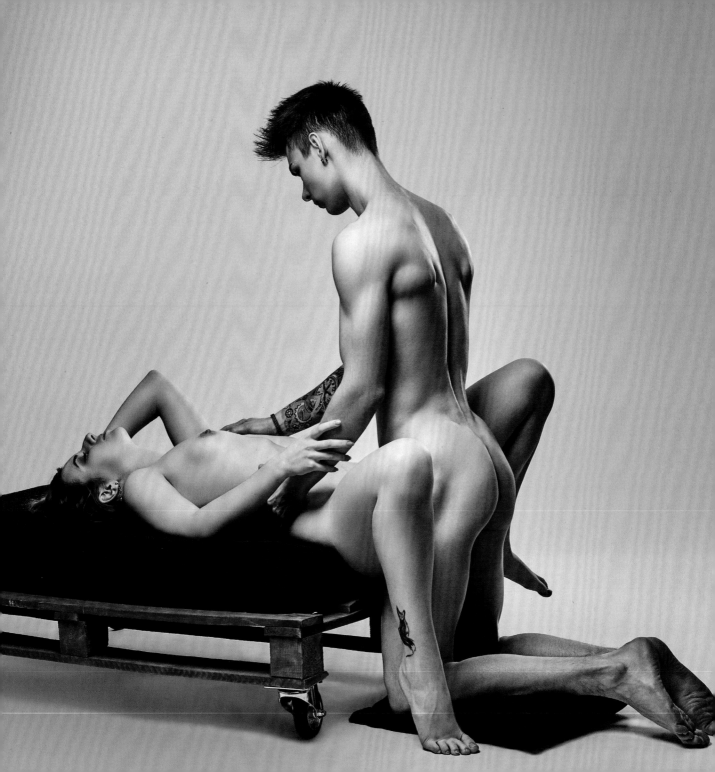

BUTTERFLY

Another variation on the standard Missionary, the Butterfly is easy to do, yet very satisfying for both male and female partners. There isn't quite as much eye contact here, but the female partner is still positioned in such a way that her lover can stimulate her nipples and clitoris with his hands.

HOW TO DO IT

The male partner is on his knees, in between his partner's legs. The female partner will support herself on a flat surface that is raised. It's easiest to achieve this position on a bed, ottoman, or coffee table. The female partner will lie back with her pelvis at the edge of the bed and her legs down and feet flat on the floor or bed frame. If the bed is very high, the male partner can stand, but a lower bed will work better if the male partner would rather be on his knees. (Don't forget a soft pillow or rug). He can hold on to her hips for leverage and more control with thrusting.

WHERE TO DO IT

If he prefers to be on his knees, then an ottoman or coffee table works best. If he prefers to stand, then a tall bed or desk will work better.

PROPS YOU'LL

A pillow or soft mat for his knees.

DIFFICULTY LEVEL ★☆☆☆☆

HER O-METER ★★★★☆

This position is actually quite comfortable for her and allows her to experience everything more fully. This is better than basic Missionary for G-spot stimulation, and allows easy access for clitoral stimulation with fingers or a small clitoral vibrator.

HIS O-METER ★★★★☆

This sex position is comfortable for him as well, but it's not as exotic as he'd like it to be. He does however have control over his orgasm here and a great view to watch her play with her clitoris.

MAKE IT HOTTER . . .

A vibrator on her clitoris is the obvious way to spice this one up a bit, but why not take it to the next level and move this outside and do it on the hood of the car, side of the pool, or deck chair . . . Now we're talking!

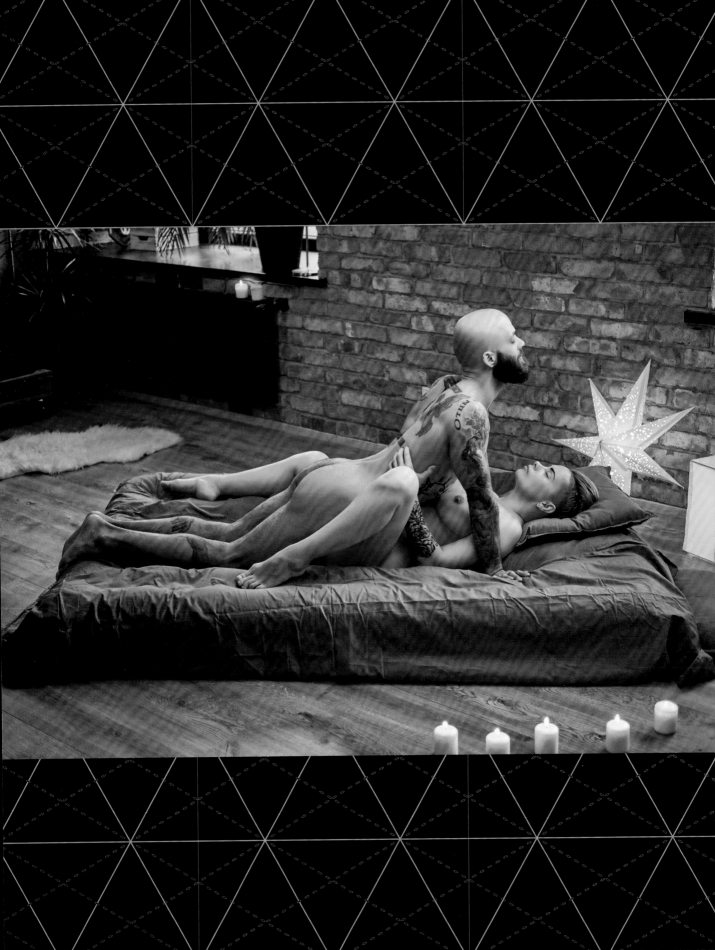

COITAL ALIGNMENT TECHNIQUE

The Coital Alignment Technique is a sex position that can be used to increase a woman's chances of orgasm in the Missionary sex position. It's a slight variation on Missionary that allows for her clitoris to receive more stimulation than in basic Missionary.

HOW TO DO IT

Assume the traditional Missionary sex position. The male partner will shift "up" slightly, while the female partner will shift her hips "down" slightly, allowing her clitoris and pubic bone to come into contact with the shaft of his penis and his pubic bone. Once you're "lined up," there's not much in and out action that's going to happen. In fact, you want to try not to break the contact between the clitoris and pubic bone as much as you can.

So how exactly does this work? Since he's not thrusting in and out per se, he's going to be using more of an up-and-down grinding motion. This will create some thrusting, but not your typical "all the way in, all the way out" sort of motion. She's going to do her best to grind against him in the same way, keeping her clitoris pressed up against him to receive the stimulation the grinding motion causes. This move actually takes some practice to really get the hang of it, but it's totally worth it when she gets to have an amazing orgasm with him on top.

WHERE TO DO IT

The bed or floor on a soft mat are best for the Coital Alignment Technique. You'll be focusing so much on lining yourselves up properly and grinding against each other that you don't want to add any logistical problems that a different location may cause.

PROPS YOU'LL NEED

A pillow under her lower back can help angle her pelvis in such a way that it's easier for her to grind against the shaft of his penis and pubic bone.

DIFFICULTY LEVEL ★★★☆☆

HER O-METER ★★★★★

Once you get this right, she's going to love the Coital Alignment Technique. Sometimes a girl just wants to lay back and let her guy take the reins, but this often means giving up the possibility that she'll have an orgasm. However, with the Coital Alignment Technique, she can feel dominated by her guy and get off at the same time.

HIS O-METER ★★★☆☆

The Coital Alignment Technique isn't quite as good for him as it is for her, because he has to move differently than he normally does. It's not a smooth in and out motion (which is what a guy really responds best to), but he's having sex so, hey, it's all good, right? Once she has a massive orgasm, he can move into a new and better position for him.

MAKE IT HOTTER . . .

Get synchronized so you're both thrusting and grinding in a smooth motion together. Gaze deeply into each other's eyes and use this opportunity to connect emotionally as well as physically. When you get good at the Coital Alignment Technique, you can easily use it to achieve simultaneous orgasm!

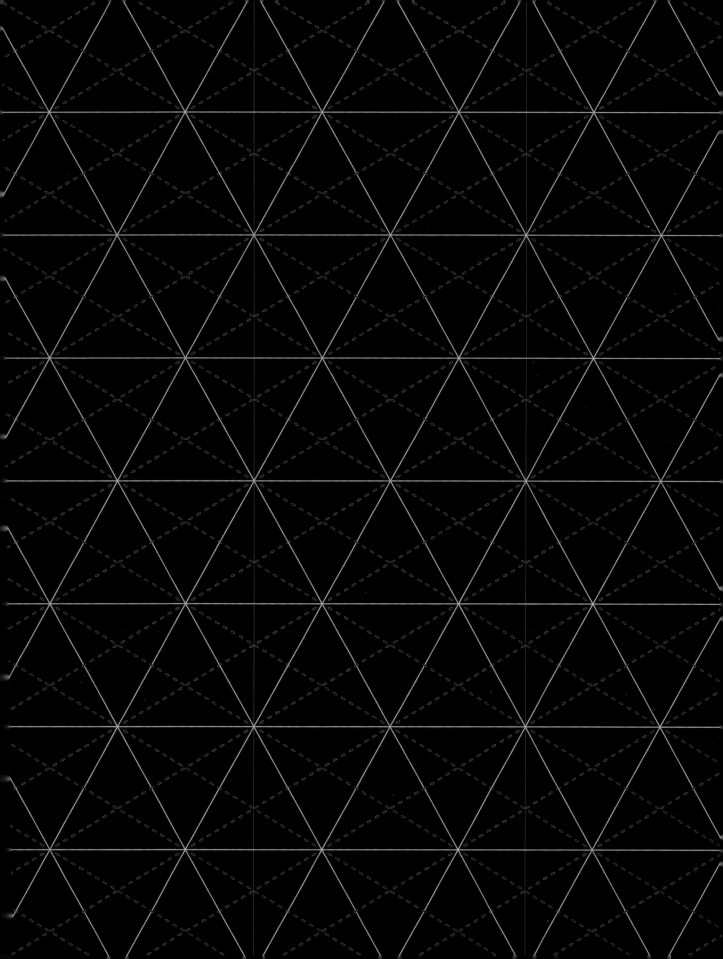

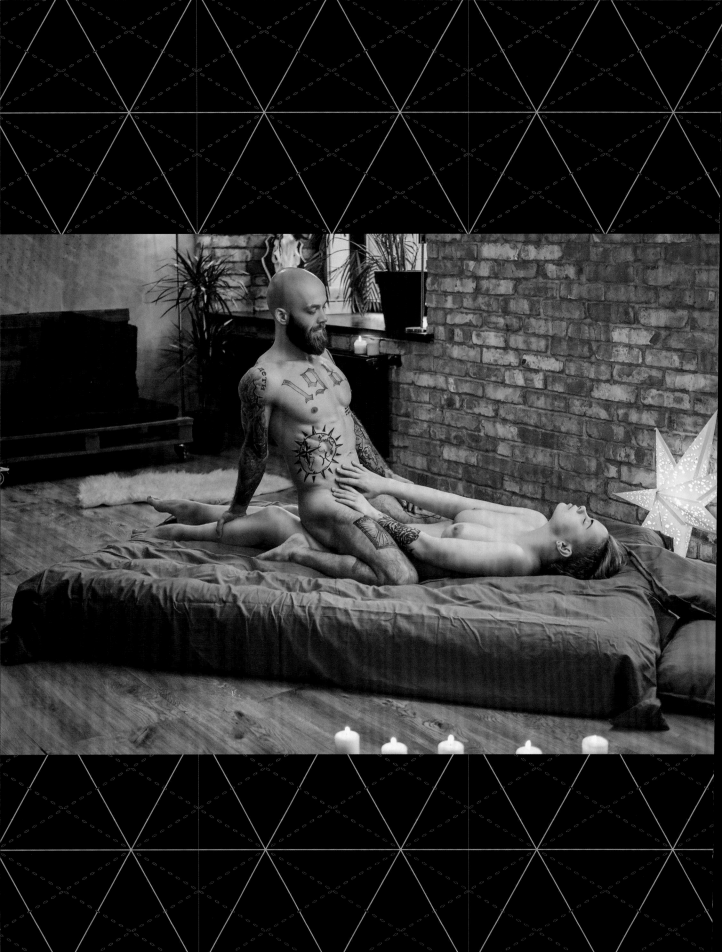

COWBOY

If you can imagine the Cowgirl sex position (see page 45), but with the man on top, you'll have the Cowboy. It's a fun twist on the Missionary, or "him on top" sex!

HOW TO DO IT

The female partner lies on her back with her legs pressed together, similar to as if she were in the traditional Missionary sex position. Her partner will then straddle her with each leg on either side of her to penetrate. He's sitting straight up, "cowboy" style. He's not used to thrusting like this, so it may take some time for him to get the hang of it.

WHERE TO DO IT

A flat surface such as the bed, sofa, or floor is best for the Cowboy sex position. This can be a fun one to do outdoors while camping or doing something else "rugged" or "outdoorsy."

PROPS YOU'LL NEED

Depending on where you do it, she may want a pillow or two under her head, or you may want to spread a blanket out first.

DIFFICULTY LEVEL ★★★☆☆

HER O-METER ★☆☆☆☆

Let's be honest here . . . unless he has a rather long penis, she is not going to get much out of this one. Because of the angle of penetration, the average length penis is not going to get enough penetration depth for her. It's a great position to try once so you can say you did, but there are many others that she will enjoy much better.

HIS O-METER ★★★☆☆

Because her legs are together, the penetration is nice and tight, even though it's not as deep as it is in other sex positions, so this is still a win for him. She can make it even better for him by squeezing her thighs together and rotating her hips slightly upward.

MAKE IT HOTTER . . .

Have some fun with this one and break out the cowboy hat and chaps. Maybe even add a bondage component and lasso her with some rope and tickle her with your spurs or a Wartenberg pinwheel.

DELIGHT

A variation on the Missionary, the Delight is simple, but both intimate and erotic. It's a perfect sex position to use if you want lots of eye contact, but it's also great if you want to get kinky and watch the action down below. You definitely want to try this one, and use it again and again!

HOW TO DO IT

This is an exceptionally easy sex position to master and is highly arousing and satisfying for both partners. The female partner simply sits on a bed or chair with her legs spread and her feet flat on the floor. The male partner gets on his knees and aligns his pelvis in between her legs for thrusting. It's simple, but both partners get an exceptional amount of pleasure from the Delight!

WHERE TO DO IT

The sofa, edge of a low bed, or chair is perfect for this position.

PROPS YOU'LL NEED

A soft blanket or pillow for his knees will make this position more comfortable for him.

DIFFICULTY LEVEL ★☆☆☆☆

HER O-METER ★★★☆☆

While this sex position allows for a fair amount of clitoral and G-spot stimulation, that's not what a woman is going to like best about the Delight. Since she is face to face with her partner, she is going to get a lot of emotional satisfaction here. It's a very intimate position, which is definitely going to be right up her alley.

HIS O-METER ★★★☆☆

A man will like any position that a woman likes, and, let's face it, guys get pleasure from almost every sex position because of the way a man derives pleasure from sex. It's not as difficult to please a man as it is a woman. This isn't one of the sex positions that will totally wow him, though.

MAKE IT HOTTER . . . . . .

For even hotter intimacy, she can lean forward and cuddle against his chest. Or, if she wants to entice her man, she can lean back and let him play with her nipples or massage her clitoris.

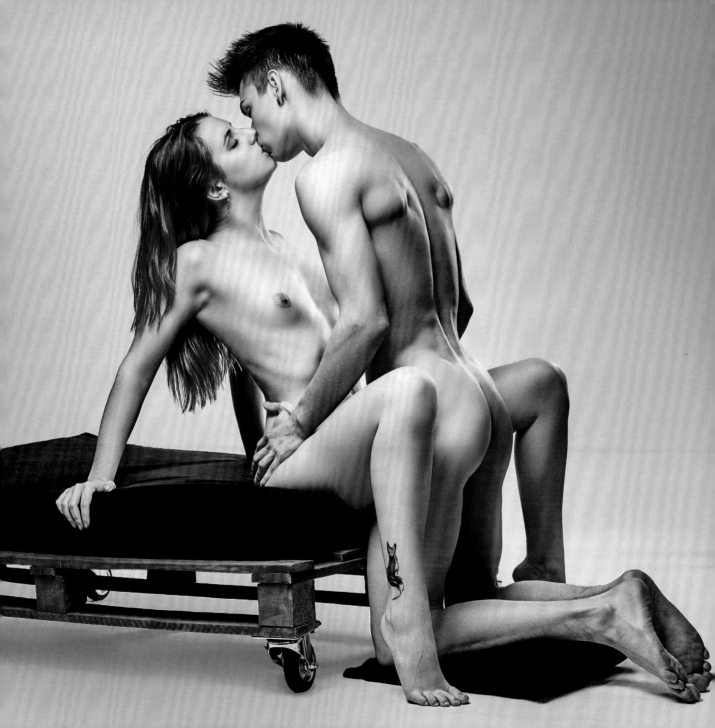

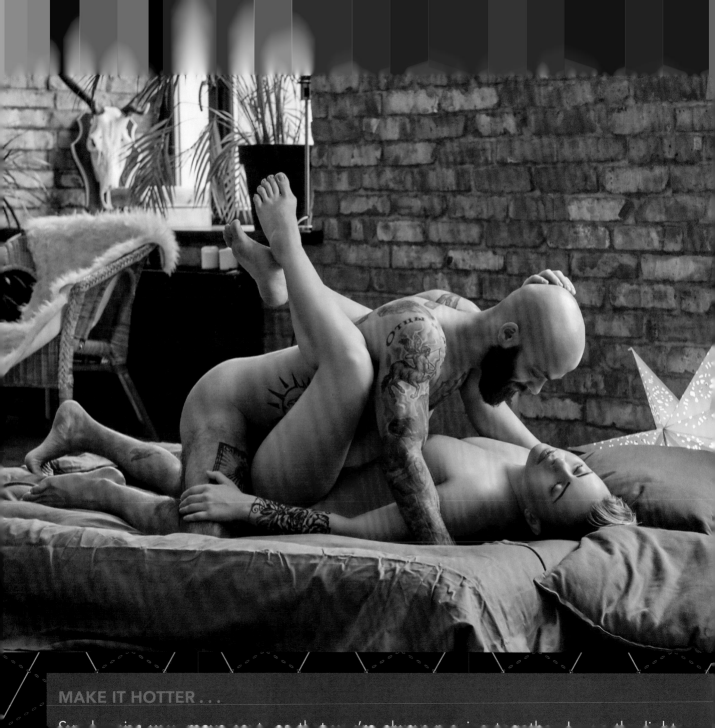

DRILL

Feel every inch of your partner during sex with the intimate, but still naughty, Drill sex position! It's a sexy twist on standard Missionary, and allows for super-deep penetration. This will result in intense g-spot stimulation for her and a mind-blowing orgasm for him! Definitely a must try.

HOW TO DO IT

The Drill is almost identical to the Deck Chair (see page 209), where the female partner is lying on her back with her partner positioned in between her legs. The main difference here is that instead of raising her legs up where her knees bend at a ninety-degree angle, the female partner wraps her legs around her partner's hips and rests her ankles against his back. In this position, his weight is more on his knees instead of his arms like standard missionary.

This position provides more physical intimacy than the Deck Chair or even the Missionary, because the position of her legs allows for only minimal separation of skin contact. Women, enjoy feeling every inch of your partner with this sex position!

WHERE TO DO IT

This versatile position can be done just about anywhere like the sofa, bed, and even the floor.

PROPS YOU'LL NEED

Any sex position where the female partner is on her back can be made more comfortable with a pillow under her lower back.

DIFFICULTY LEVEL ★☆☆☆☆

HER O-METER ★★★☆

With her legs wrapped around his lower back, she can keep herself pressed up against him and use her legs muscles to grind her pelvis against her partner's. This provides for awesome clitoral stimulation! Combined with deep penetration, a blended orgasm is definitely possible in this sex position.

HIS O-METER ★★★☆

Because he is on his knees instead of holding up the majority of his own weight with his arms (as he does in the traditional Missionary position), he can focus more on pleasure than mechanics. This is often a more natural sex position for men than the Missionary.

MEET 'N' GREET

The Meet 'n' Greet sex position puts the thrusting responsibility on the female partner, although she is still on bottom as in the traditional Missionary position. Instead of him thrusting down into her, she is pushing her pelvis up towards him and doing a majority of the movement. So hot!

HOW TO DO IT

Just as in the traditional Missionary position, the male partner is on top, and the female partner is underneath him with her legs spread on either side of her lover's hips. He is resting his weight on his knees and his hands, which are on either side of her torso. However, instead of him moving down to thrust into her, she is going to raise her hips again and again to meet him. This requires a good bit of space between both partners, so he will need to prop his torso all the way up on his hands, almost as though he's in the Doggy Style position.

WHERE TO DO IT

This position can be done on the sofa, back seat of the car, floor, bed, and anywhere else you would use the Missionary position—so long as she has a good place to put her feet and get good support so that she can thrust.

PROPS YOU'LL NEED

He may be more comfortable with a pillow under his knees if you're using the Meet 'n' Greet on a hard surface, such as the floor.

DIFFICULTY LEVEL ★☆☆☆☆

HER O-METER ★★☆☆☆

Although she has a better chance of grinding her clitoris against him, since she's in control in the Meet 'n' Greet, a woman isn't used to thrusting and may tire out quickly. She may not be able to keep this going for very long if she's not fit or strong.

HIS O-METER ★★★★☆

He digs the Meet 'n' Greet sex position because he gets to watch her thrust up towards him instead of the other way around. It's a welcome change of pace, and he totally loves the idea of her being so hot and turned on that she's got to grind against him!

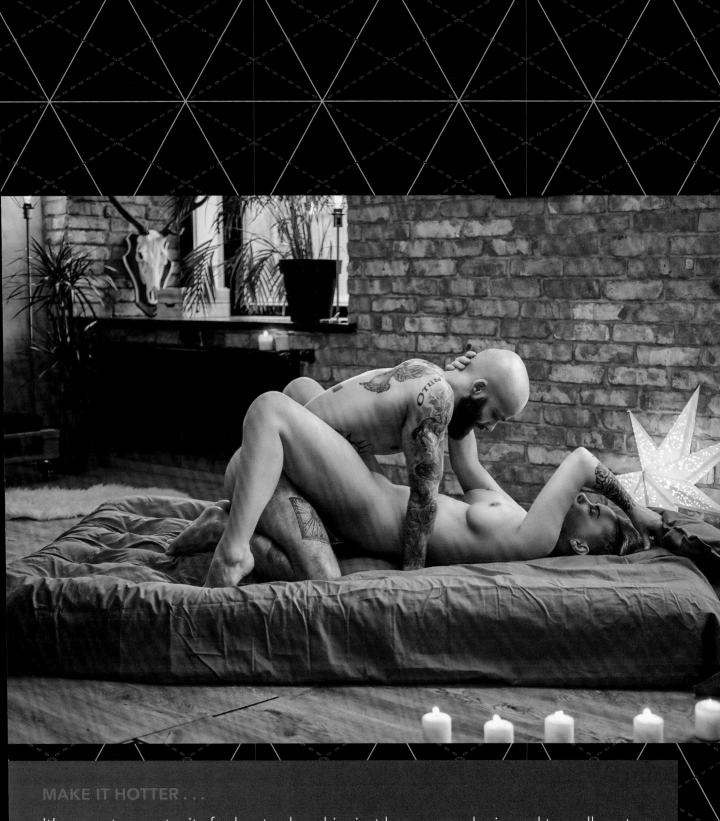

MAKE IT HOTTER . . .

It's a great opportunity for her to show him just how eager she is, and to really put on a show for him, by playing with her breasts and clitoris while he watches in ecstasy. Time to release that inner porn star!

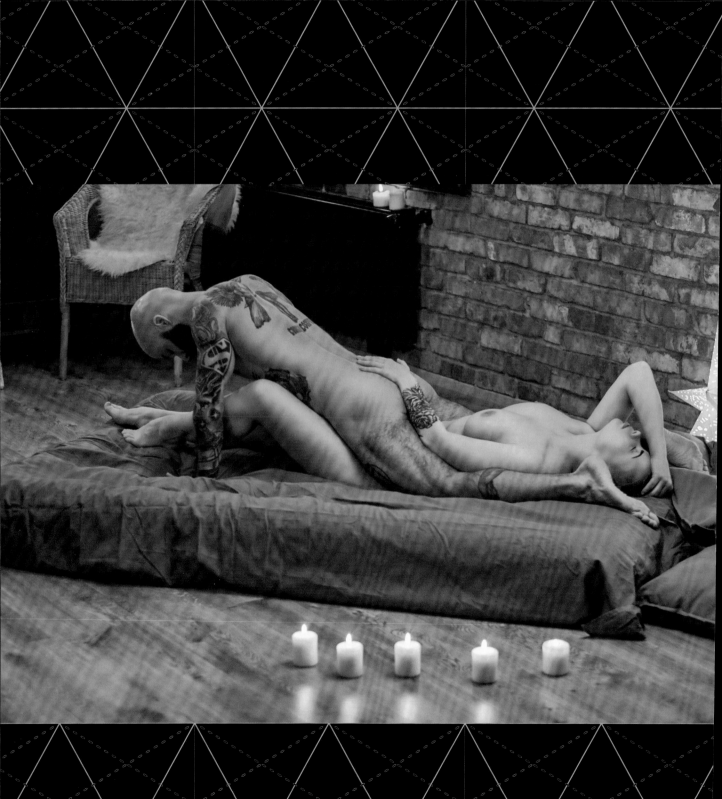

MISSIONARY REVERSED

The Missionary Reversed sex position is a fun one to try if his penis is fairly long and flexible when he's up for something a little more exotic. Some guys aren't going to dig this position because it requires them to thrust at an exceptionally odd angle, but other guys will enjoy how different this sex position is from traditional Missionary.

HOW TO DO IT

The female partner will lie flat on her back with her legs slightly spread. Her partner will then position himself on top of her, but in this position, he will be facing her feet instead of her head. His legs will also be spread enough so that they can rest on his lover's shoulders, or on either side of her head. To penetrate, he's going to push his penis downward with his fingers at the base of it, and slowly enter her. This can be quite stressful for a man's penis, so it's important to be extra lubed up and go very slowly.

WARNING: If this move hurts at all, stop immediately! Remember to thrust slowly. In rare cases, a penis can fracture when enough pressure is put on it. This usually happens suddenly, when the penis is at an odd angle and the thrusting is too fast. A penile fracture is characterized by intense, immediate pain, sudden bruising, and often an audible "fracture" sound. If this should happen, do not hesitate to seek immediate medical attention. The Missionary Reversed sex position is not dangerous in and of itself, but he can prevent any problems by communicating with his partner about any pain or discomfort he experiences and knowing when to back off.

WHERE TO DO IT

The Missionary Reversed sex position is best performed on a wide-open space like the bed or on the floor. Because you need to be focused on doing this correctly, you don't want to be crammed in the car or even on the sofa for this one.

PROPS YOU'LL NEED

Make sure to use lots of lube! You'll both need to be good and slick before attempting this position.

DIFFICULTY LEVEL ★★★★★

HER O-METER ★★★☆☆

She'll dig this sex position because it's an exotic one that doesn't involve her getting into all kinds of crazy contortionist positions. The man has to do the gymnastics on this one!

HIS O-METER ★☆☆☆☆

It's going to take a very brave man to be able to do this sex position and get off on it. The penis just isn't designed to bend this way. For him, the Missionary Reversed sex position is more about novelty than anything else.

MAKE IT HOTTER . . .

Use a liberator wedge or large pillow to make the angle of penetration better for most men.

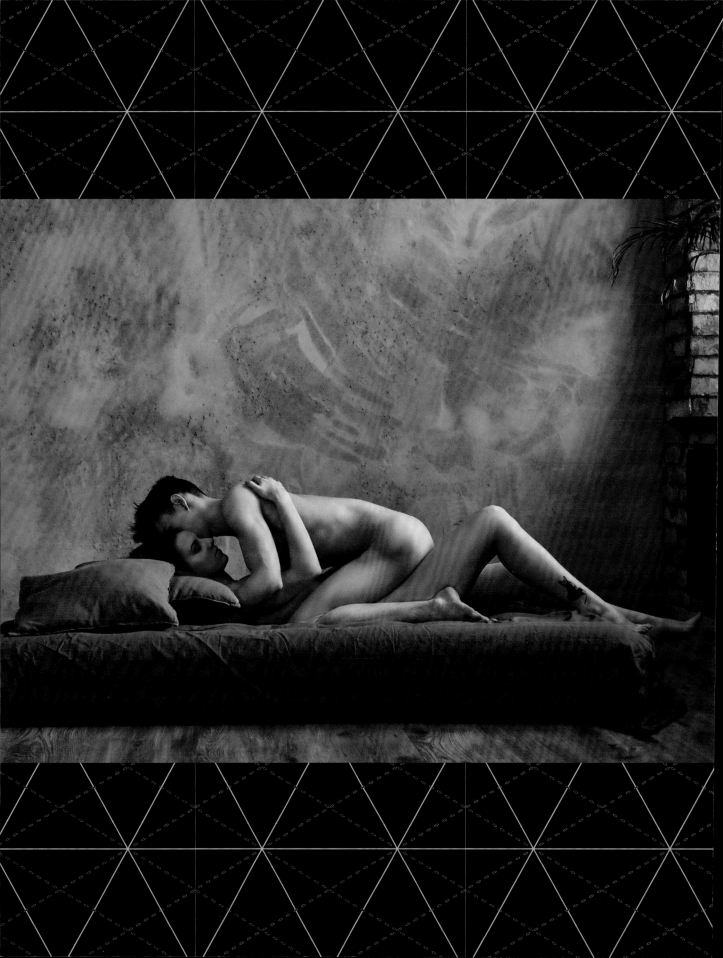

REVERSE JOCKEY

The Reverse Jockey sex position is a fun twist on the traditional Missionary that allows him to be in complete control of the thrusting and stimulation. In this position, he sits atop his partner much like a jockey sits atop a racing horse, leaning forward and downward to ride his trusty steed.

HOW TO DO IT

The female partner lies on her back, à la the traditional Missionary position. The male partner "mounts" his lady facing her head, but instead of putting his legs in between her slightly spread legs, he'll place them on either side of her. When he thrusts, he's going to lean forward and down and move his entire body instead of just his hips and buttocks.

WHERE TO DO IT

This is a great sex position to use anywhere there is a narrow space and neither partner can spread their legs wide. The bed, sofa, and back seat of the car are all great options.

PROPS YOU'LL NEED

None.

DIFFICULTY LEVEL ★☆☆☆☆

HER O-METER ★★★☆☆

The Reverse Jockey sex position is just an OK position for her. While there is good friction between her and her partner when her legs are pressed together, as well as decent clitoral stimulation, unless her partner has a longer penis, the depth of penetration may be lacking.

HIS O-METER ★★★★☆

With her legs pressed together, her vagina feels much tighter to him. Although he won't be able to penetrate as deeply here as with other sex positions, the Reverse Jockey sex position will squeeze his penis firmly, creating an entirely new sensation for him.

She can make it even better for him by squeezing her legs together and lifting her hips slightly to improve the angle of penetration.

MAKE IT HOTTER...

The Reverse Jockey sex position is an excellent "male dominant" sex position. This is a good position to tie her hands overhead and even bind her ankles together.

X MARKS THE SPOT

The X Marks the Spot sex position combines the friction of Reverse Jockey and some deeper penetration making a win for both sexes.

HOW TO DO IT AT

In the X Marks the Spot sex position, the woman's legs are squeezed together as in Reverse Jockey, but then lifted into the air and crossed at the ankle and bent toward her chest or straight up in the air. You can also slide to the edge of the bed (or desk/table) to make thrusting easier for him, and to change up the angle just a bit.

WHERE TO DO IT

On a bed, desk, or table.

PROPS YOU'LL NEED

No props are needed for this position, but a silk tie around her ankles is a fun addition.

DIFFICULTY LEVEL ★★☆☆☆

HER O-METER ★★★☆☆

She enjoys lying down and relaxing while her lover does the work here. The deeper penetration is good for G-spot stimulation. The only thing that would make this sex position better is if he could grind against her clitoris. Unfortunately, he can't because her legs are crossed.

HIS O-METER ★★★☆☆

He likes the X Marks the Spot position because it's easy on him, too. He simply gets to stand and thrust! Her crossed legs make for a tight vaginal entrance, which feels divine, but he doesn't get to see a whole lot here with her legs in the way.

MAKE IT HOTTER . . .

Start with traditional vaginal sex in Reverse Jockey, and then slide to the edge of the bed and switch to anal sex with X Marks the Spot.

Wanna take it even further? If you have a canopy bed or poster bed, take that silk tie I mentioned earlier and suspend her ankles from the top of the bed.

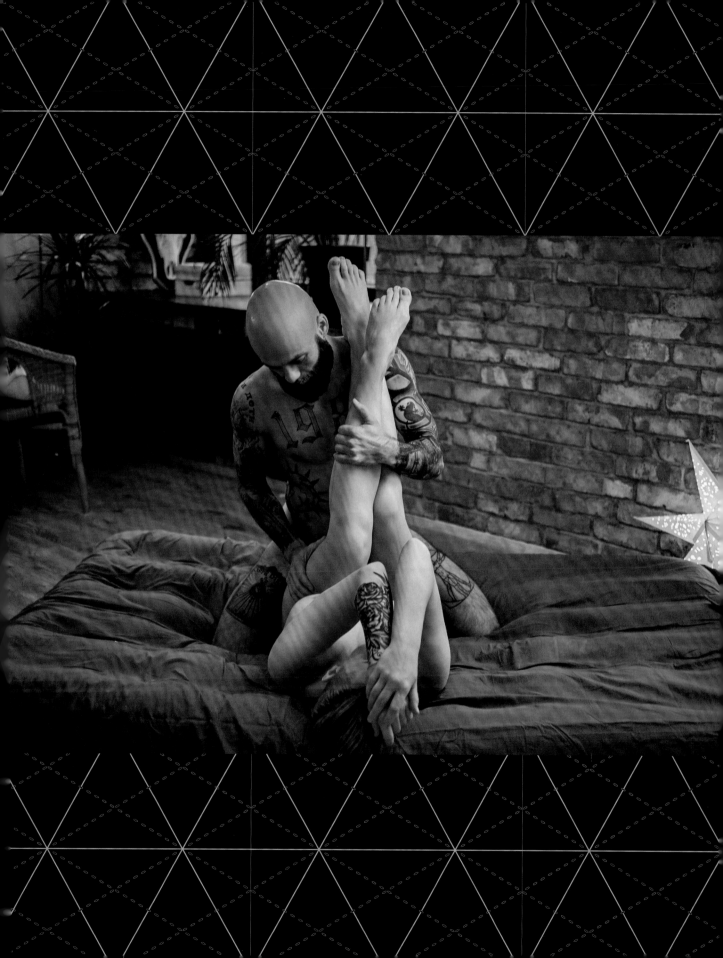

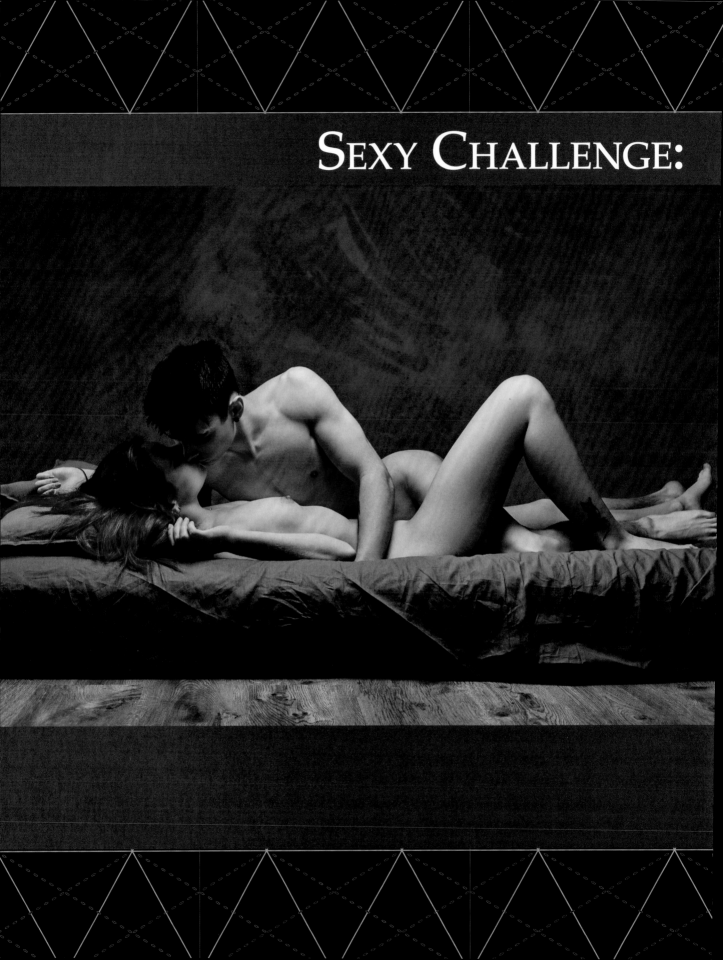

SEXY CHALLENGE:

THE MISSION

The Missionary Position—what a silly name for a sex position! A Missionary by definition is a member of a religious organization sent into an area to convert people to their religion and/or perform ministries of service, such as education, literacy, social justice, health care, and economic development. Why would you give a missionary his/her own sexual position? I am baffled.

Many people think of the Missionary Position as the most basic and the most boring sexual position ever. Why would you want that stigma attached to any sexual position? I mean think about it. Would you want to say to your partner, "Hey, want to have boring, standard sex with me?"

"Hell to the no," is what the answer should be. We have to break our minds out of the idea that the Missionary Position is basic and boring. This position, like all others, is a chance to get closer to your partner in a physical and spiritual way.

Your mission now becomes how to blow the doors off the Missionary Position stigma. You have a great start with the positions mentioned in this chapter, as they give you the base to make the Missionary Position more exciting, and more outside the box than the name might suggest. However, we always need more and more and more. So what can you do to enhance your missionary position experience? The answers are endless, and if you keep that in mind, you are open to experiencing mind-blowing sex in the Missionary Position.

The first thing is to get your mind right. Sex isn't just about getting it in, getting off, and getting out.

Sex should be about connection, and I am not saying it has to be in a committed relationship. You can have amazing, connected sex with someone and not be committed to them. The way this happens is by focusing on the other person's pleasure. Yes, you want to have pleasure too, but that will come; your main mission is making sure your partner in this sexual experience gets their pleasure.

The Missionary Position can be enhanced to the point of amazement by just focusing on some different things. First, what are your hands doing during this life-changing event? Hands, fingers, and thumbs are one of the major things that separates us from the other animals. So, what are your hands doing during sex? Are they just sitting on the bed, or maybe holding you up? Have you ever considered what the mission of your hands is during sex? One thing you can be doing with your hands that will make an amazing difference is just touching your partner's body. Reach down and grab their butt, move the hair from their face, caress their body softly, hold their hands above their head, reach down and grab their ankles; the possibilities are freaking endless. Yet most who think the missionary position is boring are just letting their hands become useless. That, my friends, is their own damn fault.

The next easy thing you can do is to adjust your body position. This can be done by the person on the bottom or the person on top. Just a little change in the angle of penetration can be the driving factor in turning the standard missionary position into a flaming love fest. Maybe you just wiggle your hips a little more from side to side; that worked wonders for Elvis. Now you can also move your body forward or backwards to change things up a bit, changing that angle of penetration, giving a vastly different feel to you and your lover.

Speed isn't going to help you at all if you are trying to make the missionary position a positive experience for everyone involved. Guys, you are not running a jackhammer, trying to break up some concrete before quitting time. Speed of thrusting can range from super slow and passionate, to hard, fast, and furious. However, keeping the throttle on one speed gets boring. Ladies, if you are on bottom during missionary position, don't think you can't control the speed. You have a lot of tools to tell your lover to speed up or slow down. Squeezing your legs together a little will give the hint to slow down, and opening your legs up and thrusting more yourself will get you the hard, fast, and furious stoke talked about above. Unless you are pressed for time and wanting a quickie, your speed should hit the highs and lows during your sexual mission.

Never ever does this book say that you have to finish in the Missionary Position if you started there, nor does it say you can't return to the missionary position after trying something different. Later in this book, you will see how you can benefit from the flow of different positions. There might be situations where it is easier for your partner to climax in the Missionary Position, and if that is the case, then the ending act might always be the Missionary Position. In return, many times it is easy to get started in the Missionary Position and get things warmed up nicely before moving on to another more taxing position. Missionary does not mean mandatory, so feel free to experiment and grow your knowledge of what brings you pleasure.

As we close here, let me just say that your mission in the Missionary Positions isn't about getting to the finish line first. Actually, if you get to the finish line first all the time, your partner might have some issues with that. Your mission should be to uncover the most amount of pleasure you can, for your partner, and in turn, for yourself. The mission in your sex life doesn't have a set course! You have to adjust and move to get the most out of every situation, and the Missionary Position is not different. While many people think of it as the standard for sex, the Missionary Position can be as hot or even hotter than any other position you can think of. Now your mission is to see just how hot you can make it.

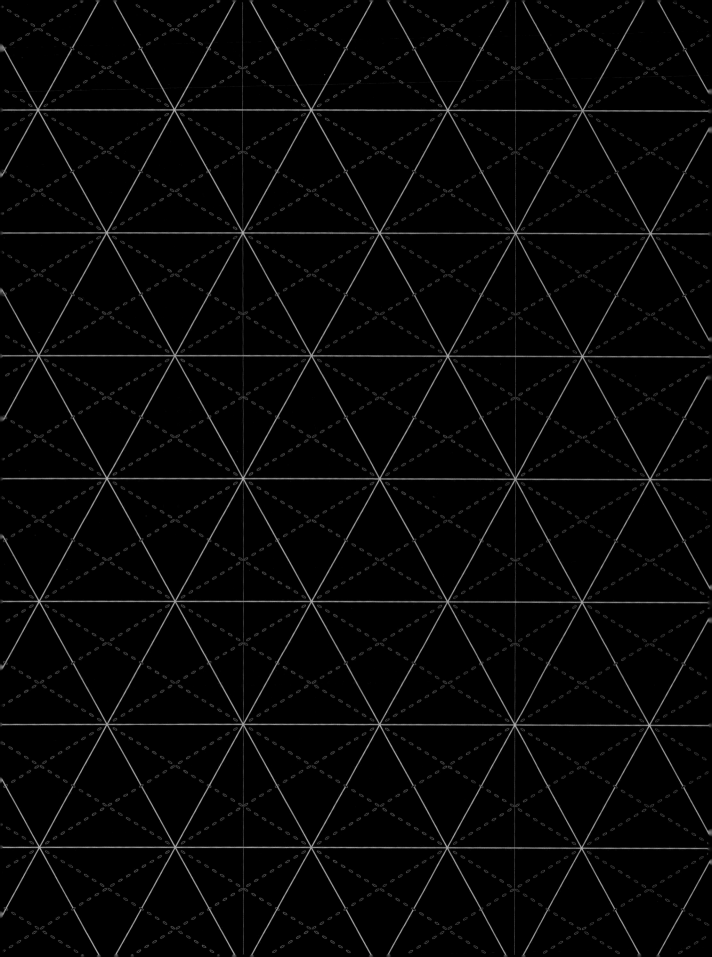

CHAPTER 3: WOMAN-ON-TOP SEX POSITIONS

AMAZON

The Amazon sex position is an exotic form of Woman on Top that's easy for her, but a bit difficult for him if he's less flexible or has a bigger belly.

HOW TO DO IT

The male partner lies on his back and raises his legs, bringing his knees up to his chest with his legs parted. The female partner then straddles his groin with his knees in front of her and his legs wrapped around her waist, with his feet at her back. The Amazon sex position puts the female partner in total control of the thrusting, but it can be a bit difficult due to the angle at which his penis must bend to enter her.

WARNING: If this is at all uncomfortable or painful for the male partner, stop immediately! Many men aren't flexible enough in the penis to pull this move off, and that's okay. The penis can actually fracture, so go slowly, and, if there is any discomfort, stop and find another sex position to try.

WHERE TO DO IT

The bed, floor, or even the back of the SUV.

PROPS YOU'LL NEED

Place a pillow under his head for comfort.

DIFFICULTY LEVEL ★★★★★

HER O-METER ★★★☆☆

The Amazon sex position is less satisfying for her than the traditional Woman-on-Top sex position because there isn't much clitoral contact here, but the dominant woman will enjoy the control over thrusting that this position affords. G-spot orgasms can be had in the Amazon sex position, but she must be careful not to ride him too hard or put too much stress on his penis since it is bent at such an odd angle.

HIS O-METER ★☆☆☆☆

He can get off in this sex position, but it may not be easy for him. He also may not be able to get into this position comfortably at all, so the only thing you can do is try it and see how it works for you.

MAKE IT HOTTER . . .

If he enjoys a prostate massage, she can reach around and play with his anus during lovemaking for an explosive orgasm. If she can't reach around very well, a small butt plug or string of anal beads could be another option.

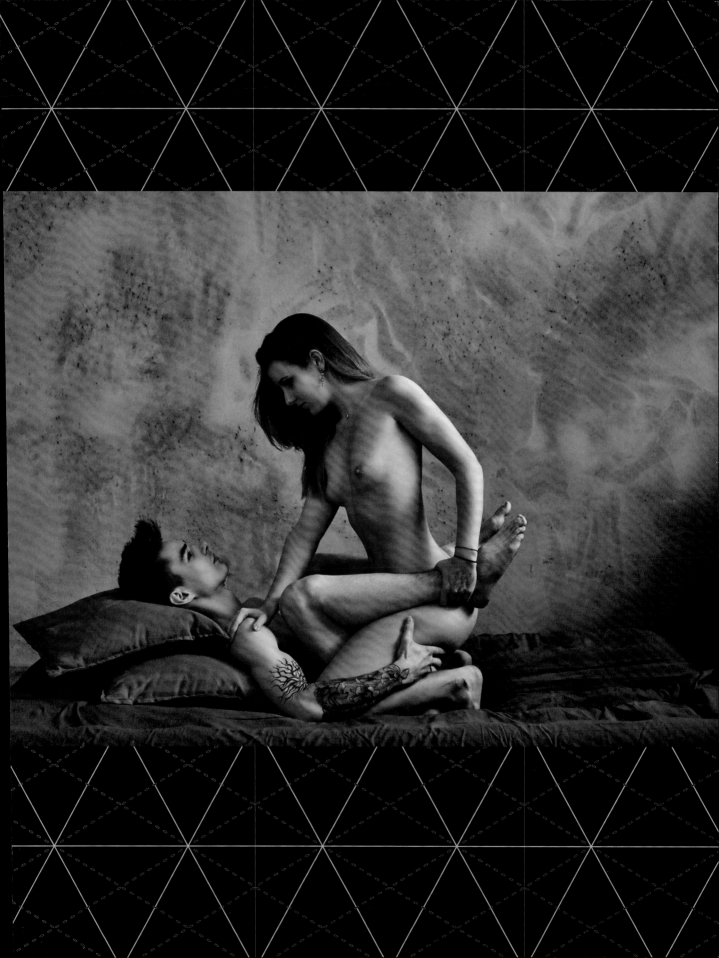

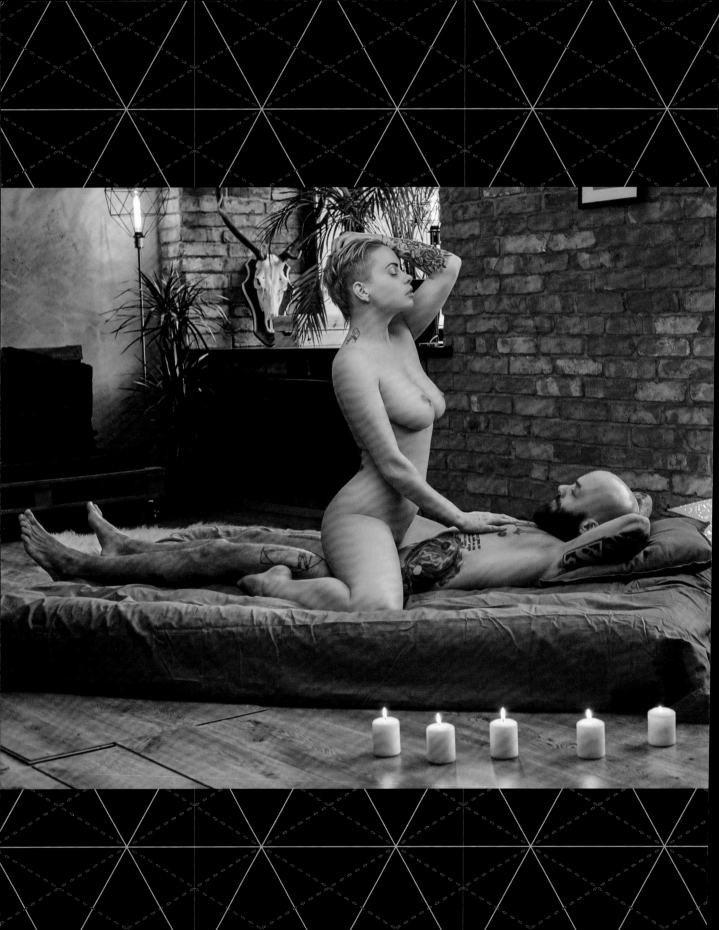

COWGIRL

The Cowgirl sex position is by far the most conducive to female orgasms, and many women can only orgasm in this position. Guys love it, too, because they get to sit back and relax while their girls take care of most of the thrusting action. This is a must-have sex position in your repertoire.

HOW TO DO IT

The Cowgirl sex position is a favorite among women! It's also known as the "Woman-on-Top" sex position. The male partner lies flat on his back (like the woman does in standard Missionary), and the female partner straddles his pelvis with her legs on either side of him, resting her weight on her knees. He can bend his knees some to help support her, or he can leave his legs lying flat on the bed. She can sit straight up, but it is more common for women to lean forward some for more clitoral stimulation.

WHERE TO DO IT

The sofa, bed, floor, or car—any reasonably flat surface will do for the Cowgirl.

PROPS YOU'LL NEED

A soft blanket or pillow to go under her knees will really help!

DIFFICULTY LEVEL ★☆☆☆☆

HER O-METER ★★★★★

The Cowgirl sex position allows a woman to control almost everything about sex—the speed and depth of penetration, as well as the angle. She can change any one of these things to better facilitate an orgasm, and this makes it much easier for her to achieve the big O. Because this sex position offers such excellent G-spot and clitoral stimulation, many women can have blended orgasms!

HIS O-METER ★★★★☆

If she's getting off, he's getting off. He really loves watching her do her thing, so this sex position gives him a great show. He really digs her riding him and using his body to get herself off.

MAKE IT HOTTER . . .

If she's sitting straight up, he's got a much better view, and she can touch herself while having sex to give him the ultimate show!

HOT SEAT

The Hot Seat sex position is a combination between Woman on Top and rear entry. It's perfect for when you're craving something a little naughty, but not too difficult to do.

HOW TO DO IT

The male partner sits with his knees bent and his feet flat on the floor, supporting his torso on either a pillow or two, or with his elbows. The female partner lowers herself onto her lover facing away from him, with her back to him and her legs bent in a similar way to his. Her hands are on his hips (not his stomach) to allow her to bear her own weight and use her muscles for thrusting and movement. You may only be able to achieve a grinding or rocking movement in this position, but many couples will enjoy how slow and sensual it is.

WHERE TO DO IT

The Hot Seat sex position is great for the sofa or a sturdy reclining chair, although it can also be done on the bed with pillows under the male partner for support.

PROPS YOU'LL NEED

A clitoral vibrator is a great addition to increase the intensity.

DIFFICULTY LEVEL ★★★☆☆

HER O-METER ★★★☆☆

Her arms can get plenty tired in the Hot Seat sex position, and there's little clitoral action going on here. However, the angle of penetration is such that it affords excellent G-spot stimulation! She may be able to coax herself to orgasm here, especially if she reaches down and stimulates her clitoris with her hand or a sex toy.

HIS O-METER ★★★☆☆

He enjoys being "ridden" in the Hot Seat sex position, but there's really nothing for him to look at other than her back. Since guys are visual creatures, they need to be able to see what is going on to really get off. But that doesn't mean this position is a total bummer for him.

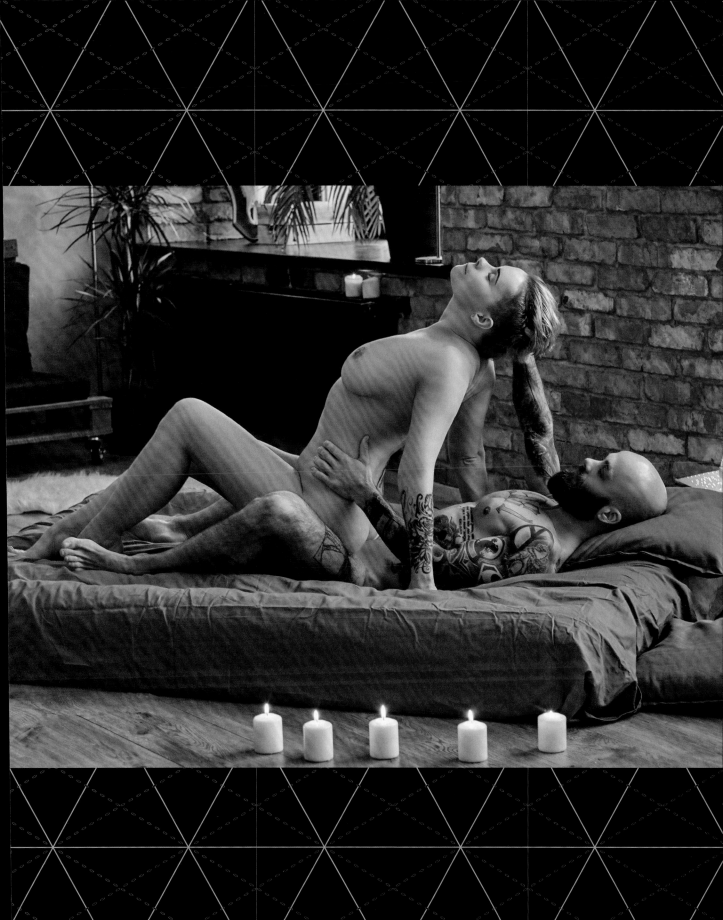

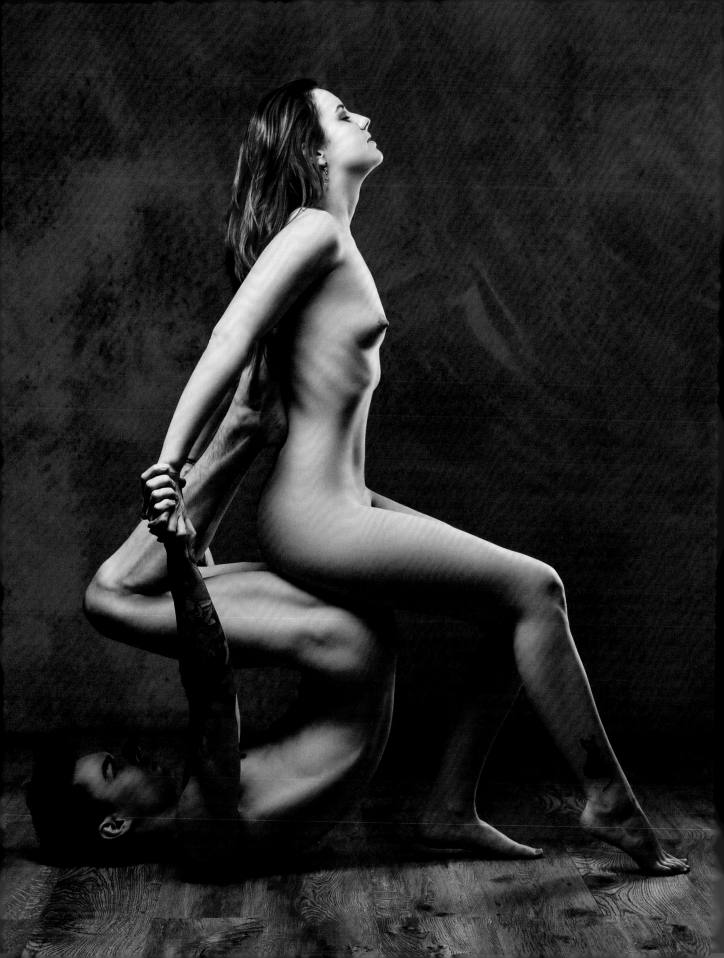

MAKE IT HOTTER . . .

Take it up a level and move into Hot Seat Advanced. To get into this position, he rolls up onto his shoulders and she takes her seats again. If you have the athletic ability, this can be an excellent position. Try it facing a wall, where he can rest his butt on the wall and she can hold onto the wall to better facilitate thrusting in this challenging position.

CRAB

The Crab sex position is a unique Woman-on-Top sex position that gives the male partner quite a show during lovemaking, even if it is a little awkward for him to do.

HOW TO DO IT

The male partner lies on his back with his legs spread a little, and the female partner sits on top of him, with her feet facing him. She can lean back and grab on to his feet to help with thrusting, or she can use her legs, which are bent so that her feet rest flat on the floor or bed on either side of her partner's torso. Although the Crab sex position allows the male partner to view penetration, it can be a difficult sex position for him to master because his penis is bent at an odd angle. It's not impossible though, because men who have a flexible penis will likely enjoy this sex position.

WARNING: If you feel discomfort or pain, stop immediately! Because the penis is bent at an unnatural angle, pain or discomfort typically signals that your body isn't ready to do that yet. Play it safe, and find another sex position if you find this one hurts.

WHERE TO DO IT

The Crab sex position can be done on any flat surface, but you'll both probably appreciate the comfort of a bed.

PROPS YOU'LL NEED

He may want a pillow or two under his head to help support him, so he can see the action if he's not propped up on his elbows.

DIFFICULTY LEVEL ★★★☆☆

HER O-METER ★★★☆☆

While the Crab sex position doesn't afford her much clitoral stimulation on its own, her partner can easily reach for her clitoris and stimulate it during thrusting with his hands (which will make the show even more fun!). She may really enjoy the dominance of this sex position, even if getting the hang of thrusting is a little challenging.

HIS O-METER ★★★☆☆

If he can get into the Crab sex position comfortably, it's likely to be an exceptionally enjoyable position for him because he can see everything that is going on. However, if it is uncomfortable or his penis isn't flexible, he's not likely to enjoy it. Go slow until you get the hang of how to thrust and move in this sex position.

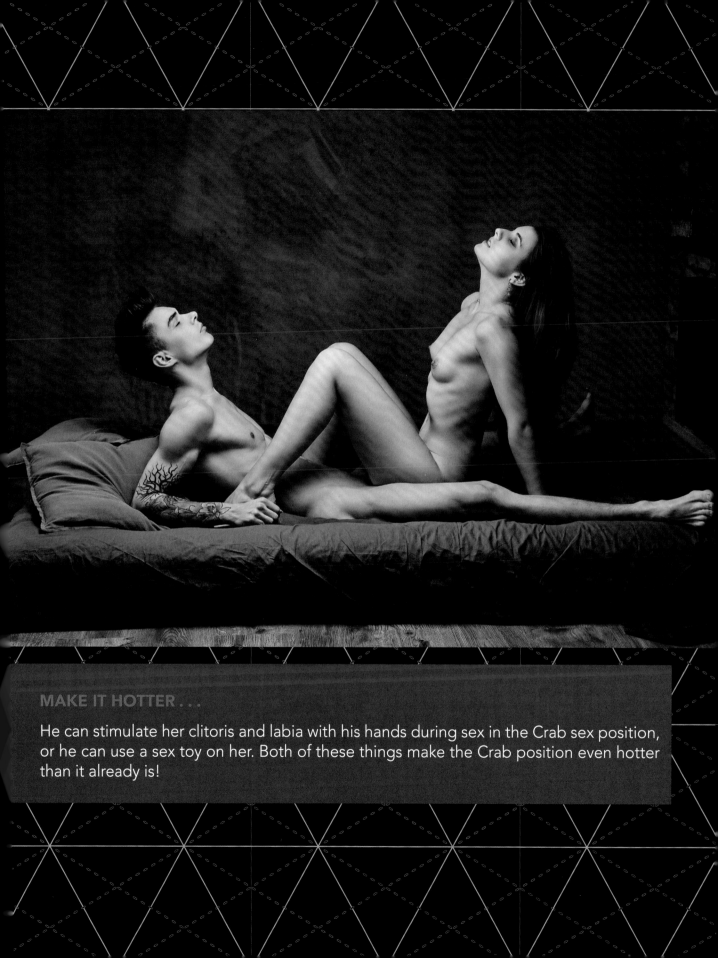

MAKE IT HOTTER . . .

He can stimulate her clitoris and labia with his hands during sex in the Crab sex position, or he can use a sex toy on her. Both of these things make the Crab position even hotter than it already is!

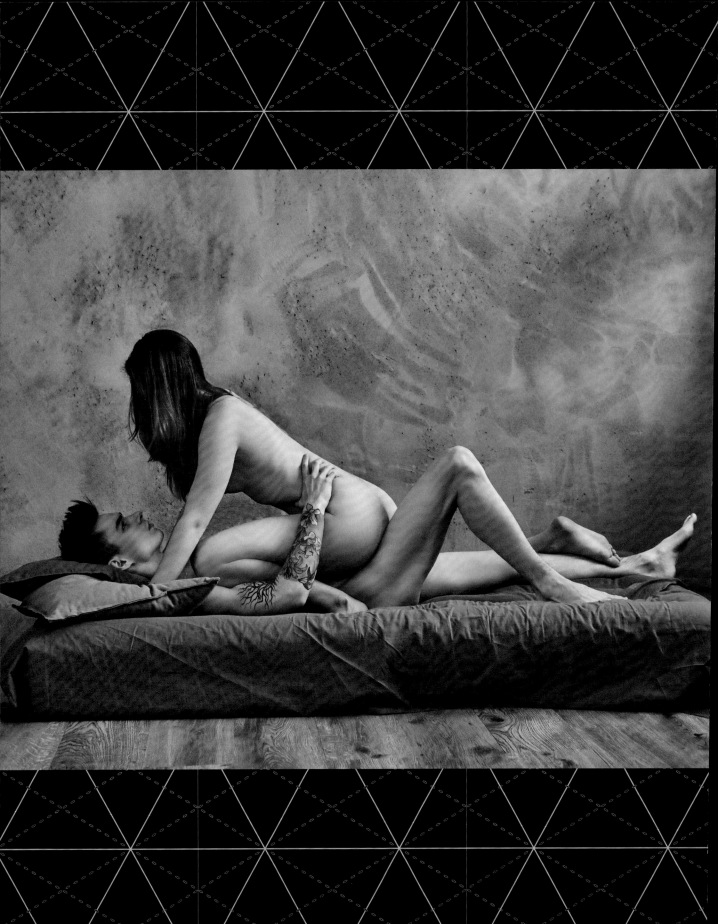

LUNGE

The Lunge sex position is a fun twist on Woman on Top that allows for super-deep penetration. The only trick is that the female partner must be quite flexible.

HOW TO DO IT

The male partner lies on his back with his legs spread open a little past shoulder width. The female partner begins to come up in between his legs (almost as though this was Missionary, but with her playing the role of the man), and raises one leg up, hooking it around his hip, while resting her foot on the bed and against the outside of his buttocks. The other leg is still straight and positioned between his legs, flush with the bed. The Lunge sex position gets its name because it looks like the female is doing a "lunge" type of stretch as she lowers herself onto his penis.

WHERE TO DO IT

This is one you'll want to do in a bed or on the floor. You'll want all the comfort and space you can get here.

PROPS YOU'LL NEED

A pillow for him is nice, especially if he wants his head supported so he can see more of the action.

DIFFICULTY LEVEL ★★★★☆

HER O-METER ★★★☆☆

Although the Lunge sex position allows for fairly good clitoral friction and excellent deep penetration and G-spot stimulation, it can be quite difficult for a woman to get into and stay in—and even harder for her to figure out how to thrust in. She must be pretty flexible to pull this off comfortably, but if she can, the mix between clitoral friction and deep G-spot stimulation can result in some powerful orgasms.

HIS O-METER ★★★★☆

He likes the Lunge sex position because it allows him to lie back, relax, and enjoy her taking control. He also likes to watch her here, because if she lifts the bent leg ever so slightly, it provides him with a pretty decent view of the action.

MAKE IT HOTTER . . .

He can reach up and play with her nipples in the Lunge sex position, or if both partners are feeling extra naughty, he can reach around to her backside for some anal play, since the position of her legs leaves her anal area exposed.

REARVIEW MIRROR

If you're looking for an exotic-yet-easy rear-entry sex position, the Rearview Mirror will definitely fit the bill. It's fun to try!

HOW TO DO IT

The male partner sits on a surface like the floor or bed with his legs stretched out, and spread apart slightly so his lover can fit in between them. The female partner then lies on her stomach, in between his legs, with her head facing his feet, and her legs spread wide enough to allow his torso in between them. It may take some practice to align your groins perfectly, but it is possible!

In this position, he won't be able to do much of the thrusting, so she will be in charge of the rhythm and depth of the thrusts. The Rearview Mirror Sex Position is similar to the Reverse Cowgirl sex position, so if this one feels awkward, try that one first.

WHERE TO DO IT

Since a fair amount of space is required for this position, you'll want to do it on the floor or the bed. A sofa or another narrow space just isn't going to work out as well.

PROPS YOU'LL NEED

A blanket or thick towel will make this position more comfortable on the floor.

DIFFICULTY LEVEL ★★★☆☆

HER O-METER ★★★☆☆

While the Rearview Mirror sex position is fairly comfortable for her, the angle of penetration may be a bit awkward at first, as will getting the hang of thrusting. In this sex position, it's less actual "thrusting," and more of a rocking, grinding motion. This, however, can help stimulate her clitoris for more orgasm potential!

HIS O-METER ★★★☆☆

He likes the view in the Rearview Mirror sex position; however, it may be a bit of an awkward angle for his penis to bend. If he's very flexible in the penis, it may not be a big issue, and he can enjoy the rocking and grinding while he gets to watch the action!

WARNING: If there is any discomfort in this sex position, stop immediately! The angle of penetration might cause the penis to bend in a different direction than you're used to. This can take some adjusting to, so go slowly, and if it's uncomfortable or painful at any point, stop and try a different sex position.

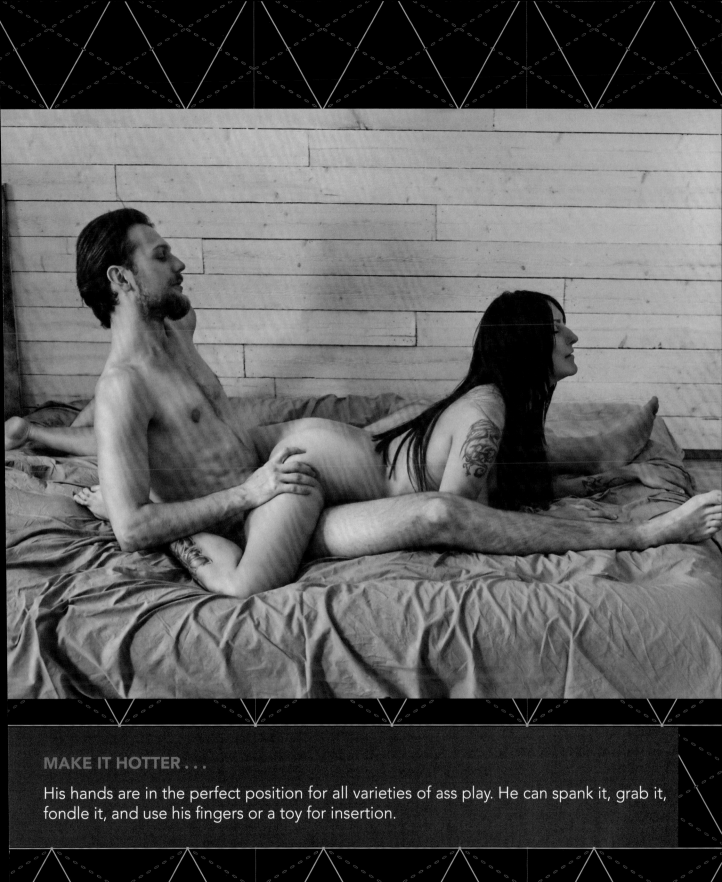

MAKE IT HOTTER . . .

His hands are in the perfect position for all varieties of ass play. He can spank it, grab it, fondle it, and use his fingers or a toy for insertion.

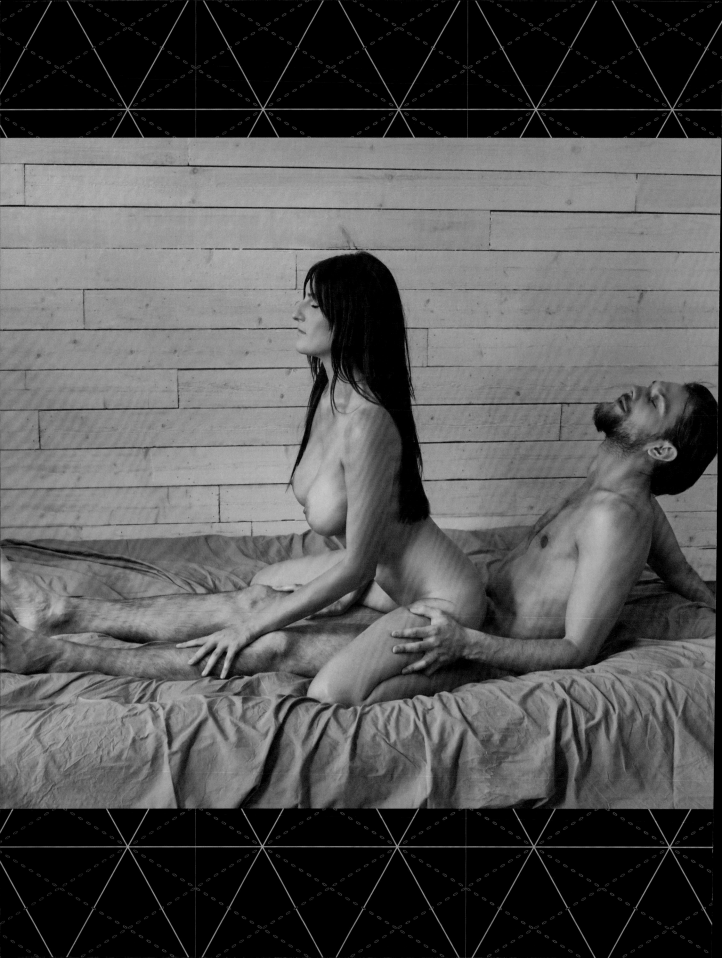

REVERSE COWGIRL

The Reverse Cowgirl is one of the best sex positions for a guy, because he gets quite the view while she rides him up and down. It's not quite as orgasmic as the Cowgirl is for a woman, but it's a little kinkier and can be a lot of fun for both partners.

HOW TO DO IT

This is a good "Woman-on-Top" sex position, and it's almost identical to the Cowgirl, with one exception. Instead of straddling her lover while facing him, the female partner straddles him facing his feet, again with one leg on either side of him with her weight resting on her knees. This position is also known as the "Rodeo."

WHERE TO DO IT

Try this one on the bed, sofa, floor, or back seat of the car—anywhere you have space to lie down!

PROPS YOU'LL NEED

None.

DIFFICULTY LEVEL ★☆☆☆☆

HER O-METER ★★★☆☆

The Reverse Cowgirl sex position isn't as powerful for a woman as the Cowgirl is. While she still gets to control the speed, depth, and angle of penetration, because she's facing her lover's feet, his anatomy doesn't line up to her hot spots as well. It's still possible for her to get G-spot stimulation from his penis, but not as easily because the penis is rubbing the wall of her vagina that her G-spot isn't on. She can get some clitoral stimulation if she leans forward far enough to rest her clitoris against his scrotum, but he may not like intense grinding against his tender bits.

HIS O-METER ★★★★★

Men really love the Reverse Cowgirl sex position. It gives them as much visual stimulation as many rear-entry sex positions do, but it combines the excitement of her controlling the action. If a woman wants to surprise her man with a super-hot sex position, the Reverse Cowgirl is the way to go.

MAKE IT HOTTER . . .

This is a wonderful position for her to reach down and massage his prostate!

SEATED SCISSORS

The Seated Scissors sex position is a fun position that allows her to be on top, and get great clitoral stimulation, too.

HOW TO DO IT

The male partner lies on his back on a bed and spreads his legs with one knee bent. His partner gets on top of him and intertwines her legs with his. She is facing away from him and straddling his thigh so that her groin is pressed against his leg and he is able to penetrate her. It's similar to Reverse Cowgirl (see page 57), but she is riding his leg instead of his torso.

WHERE TO DO IT

The Seated Scissors sex position requires so much space that you're better off doing it on the bed. While the floor will work, the bed is certainly the most comfortable option. If you do decide to do it on the floor, make sure you have plenty of blankets and pillows! It's also a fun sex position to do outdoors on a picnic blanket, if you have enough privacy!

PROPS YOU'LL NEED

Blankets and pillows, depending on where you are.

DIFFICULTY LEVEL ★★☆☆☆

HER O-METER ★★★★☆

She likes the Seated Scissors sex position because it's exceptionally easy for her to get clitoral stimulation. She can grind her clitoris up against his thigh, and with some lube, it can feel absolutely fantastic. And unlike traditional Scissors (see page 191), she is in full control of the movement.

HIS O-METER ★★★☆☆

He likes watching her enjoy this one! Because she is in control, it may not be as orgasmic for him as some of the other positions.

MAKE IT HOTTER...

Put a few drops of lube on the inside of his thigh, where she's going to be rubbing her clitoris, for an ultra-slick, orgasmic feeling. She can also make the Joystick sex position better for him by turning around and making eye contact with him as she grinds against his thigh and fondles her own breasts.

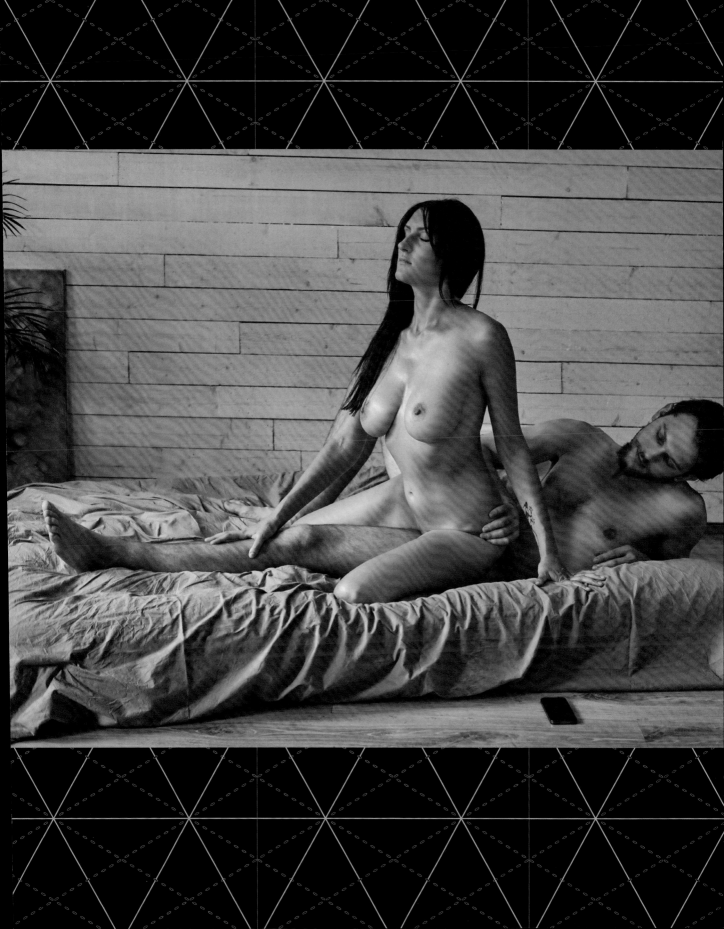

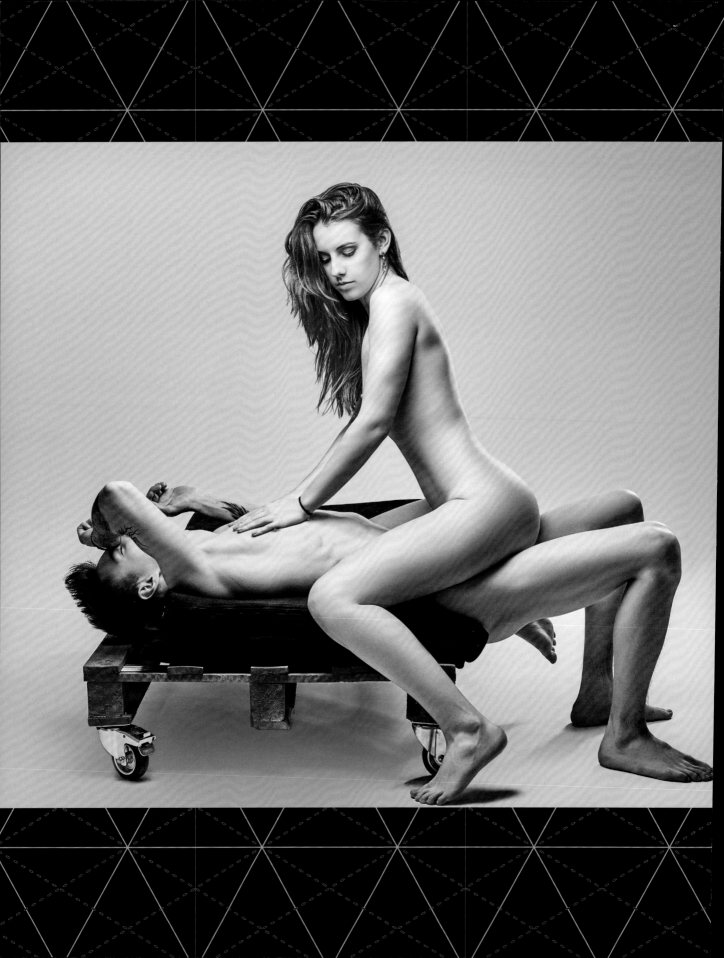

SYBIAN

Just like Sybian sex toys, the Sybian sex position allows the female partner to be in complete control, and thrust and grind herself to orgasm.

HOW TO DO IT

The male partner lies back on an ottoman or small table, with his feet flat on the floor. The chosen piece of furniture should be long enough so that his head is and hips are supported, and only his feet and legs are draped over the side. The female partner straddles his hips and lowers herself onto his penis while facing him, and uses him to grind and thrust her way to a G-spot or clitoral orgasm—or both!

WHERE TO DO IT

This one is best performed on a large ottoman or long, narrow coffee table.

PROPS YOU'LL NEED

Other than the right-size furniture, you really don't need anything extra for this one.

DIFFICULTY LEVEL ★★★☆☆

HER O-METER ★★★★★

Since she is in complete control here, she can give herself as much or as little clitoral friction as she needs to orgasm. She can also choose what depth and speed to thrust at, stimulating her G-spot in just the right way. The Sybian sex position is named after the popular Sybian sex toy, which is a mountable toy that allows a woman to ride herself to complete bliss. Doing it with a real person can be just as satisfying, if not more so!

HIS O-METER ★★★★☆

He enjoys laying back and allowing his partner to be in control every once in a while, and for guys who don't know much about how to give a woman an orgasm during intercourse, the Sybian sex position is an excellent option, since she takes the reins and is responsible for giving herself an orgasm while using his "equipment." He also enjoys the view!

MAKE IT HOTTER . . .

He is your toy in this position, so enjoy the ride and give him a good show!

SIDE SADDLE

The Side Saddle sex position is a unique twist on Woman on Top, and can be fun for both partners, but it is a little more difficult for her than it is him.

HOW TO DO IT

The male partner lies on the edge of the bed or the sofa, completely flat. The female partner stands at his hips, facing away from him, and lowers herself onto his groin, with her feet still on the floor. Her body will be perpendicular to his, and she will be facing away from him throughout lovemaking. She will use her legs and arms to push herself up and down on his penis.

WHERE TO DO IT

The Side Saddle is best performed on the sofa or the edge of the bed, but a lounge chair by the pool may be fun as well.

PROPS YOU'LL NEED

He may want a pillow, but it's not essential, especially if you're on a comfortable surface, like the sofa or bed.

DIFFICULTY LEVEL ★★★☆☆

HER O-METER ★☆☆☆☆

This can be a difficult sex position for her to master and enjoy, simply because she is responsible for all the movement during sex. The Side Saddle sex position requires substantial strength in the arms and legs, and a certain amount of stamina and endurance as well. If your leg and arm muscles aren't used to physical strain, you might feel them start to burn after just a few minutes of moving yourself up and down. However, athletic women may truly enjoy the control they have in this sex position!

HIS O-METER ★★★★☆

The Side Saddle sex position is a breeze for him, because all he's doing is laying there! He's quite comfortable here and can relax and enjoy the sensations as long as his lover can keep it up. He'll enjoy letting her "take the reins" for a little while!

MAKE IT HOTTER . . .

She can make the Side Saddle sex position more enjoyable if she thinks of her man as a "living Sybian sex toy." He is a penis for her to ride and enjoy. He, by the way, will greatly enjoy her confidence and freedom!

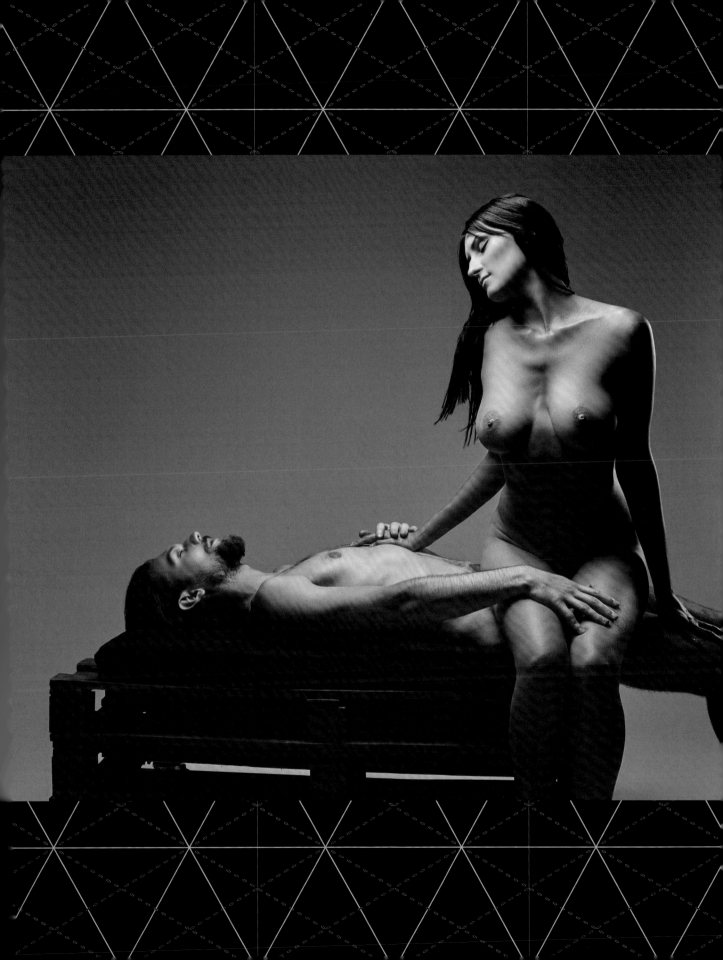

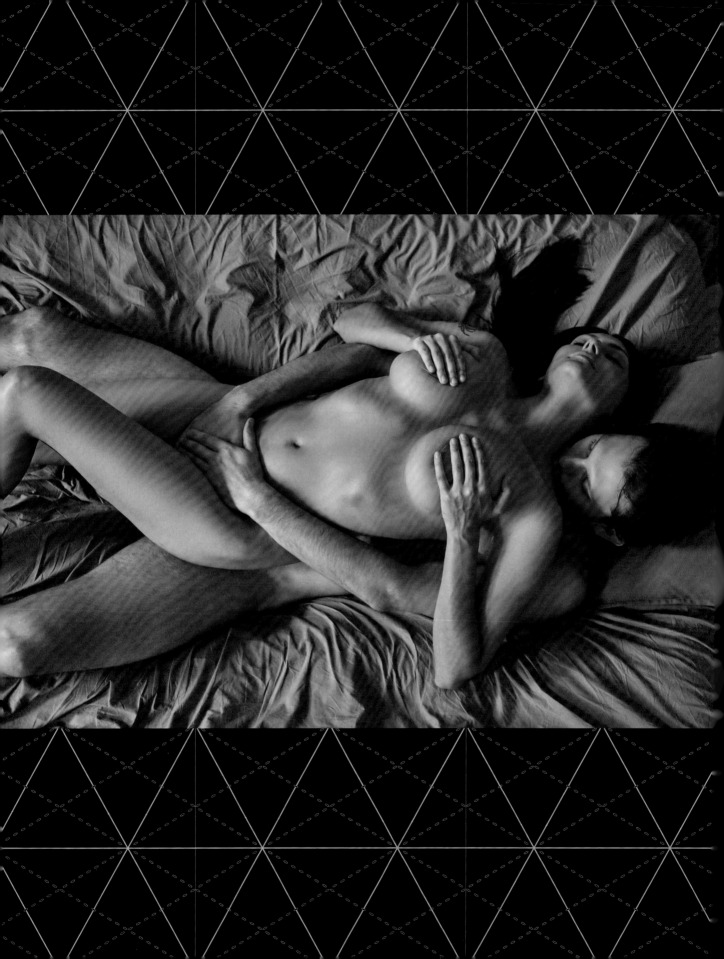

SUNNY SIDE UP

The Sunny Side Up sex position is an interesting twist on both rear entry and woman on top. She'll love this sex position as much as he does!

HOW TO DO IT

The male partner lies on a flat surface face up, and his partner lies on top of him, also face up, so her back is pressed against his torso. He enters her this way from behind, and grasps her hips to help push her up and down on top of him. This is both a somewhat exotic, yet sweet and sensual, sex position that both partners will enjoy! However, this is not a good sex position to try if the female partner is on the heavy side, because it will be much more difficult for him to stay comfortable and lift her hips up and down.

WHERE TO DO IT

The Sunny Side Up is an excellent sex position for the back seat of the car or the sofa, if you're looking for something other than your traditional Missionary to try in these places.

PROPS YOU'LL NEED

He will be very grateful for a pillow under his head!

DIFFICULTY LEVEL ★★★☆☆

HER O-METER ★☆☆☆☆

She loves the intimacy of the Sunny Side Up sex position, and enjoys it fairly well, but it's not particularly orgasmic for her unless her lover reaches around and stimulates her clitoris, or she does it herself.

HIS O-METER ★★★☆☆

His arms may tire some from lifting his partner's hips up and down to facilitate thrusting, but he will enjoy the closeness and uniqueness that the Sunny Side Up sex position has to offer. It's definitely on his "must-try" list! He'll really enjoy reaching up and fondling her breasts as she grinds against him.

MAKE IT HOTTER . . .

This is a great sex position for the adventurous couple who enjoys anal sex, because it provides a more intimate way to engage in anal than traditional anal sex positions like Doggy Style. She can make the Sunny Side Up sex position super hot by using a clitoral vibrator on herself while she grinds against her lover's groin!

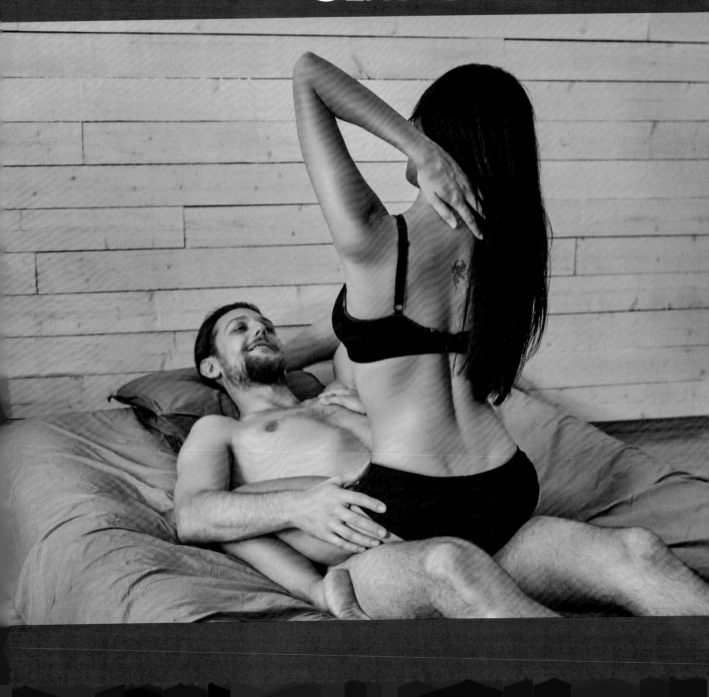

THE GODDESS ON HER CHARIOT

Women are amazing, and beautiful, and they all possess within them the power of all the Goddesses that have ever been. The Woman-on-Top positions allow the Goddess to take control of her pleasure, but that does not mean that the male remains calm and passive in the process. In this Sexy Challenge dedicated to the Woman-on-Top Positions, the male becomes not only the vessel of pleasure, but an active participant, too.

The male prepares for himself to become the chariot to carry his Goddess to pleasure. He picks the position from this chapter of the book, making sure he is erect and ready to pleasure the Goddess. As the Goddess approaches, he offers his magical member to her for her pleasure. As she approaches and positions herself, the male begins the tantalization of the skin.

The male allows his hands to explore the Goddess's sensual skin. Using random patterns of his hands, which are touching from light to firm, the male's goal here is to send sensation through the Goddess to help her open up and receive the erect penis which is the chariot that will carry her on the ride of pleasure. The male will continue stroking and fondling the Goddess, until she is fully prepared to mount the erect penis.

Now a normal Goddess riding upon her chariot is a calm sensation and a gentle ride. This ride is going to be more of a roller-coaster ride of sensual excitement. While the male encourages the Goddess to move and grind to her enjoyment on his member, the chariot should now come alive to aid and assist in the climax of the goddess.

The chariot should continue the assault with the movement of the hands. This should get even more aggressive as the pleasure in the Goddess continues to mount. The male should watch and see what seems to add to the pleasure of the Goddess. For example, does she respond to the caressing, squeezing, or grabbing her breasts, buttocks, or other areas of her body? Also consider pinching the nipples, caressing the breasts, fondling her feet, etc.

The Goddess must remember that she is in control of this chariot. She is the focal point in this parade of pleasure, and should assume that role. She should instruct the chariot driver of what she desires. If she wants the chariot to move faster or slower, or if she wants the chariot to become a bucking bronco, all she needs to do is ask. The Goddess also can use her hands either for balance, or to help her along on her journey of pleasure. She can touch her male counterpart on the areas that turn her on, by placing them on her partners chest, arms, or even reaching around to play with his genitals, while she enjoys the ride.

As the Goddess approaches climax, the male partner might need to assist her in reaching the pleasure plateau. The male can thrust his hips in various motions that could help send her over the edge. He could also draw her hands down to encourage her to add pleasure to herself as she rides her chariot. As she begins to climax, the male should grab her and hold her onto the chariot. The male can hold her by the waist, grab her forearms and pull them down, or reach up and hold on to her shoulders, so she cannot escape the sensations she is about to experience.

After the major climax, the male should release the Goddess from his grip and allow her to finish and reach the enjoyment of coming down off the organic mountain she has just climbed. The male should rejoice in the fact that as the passion chariot he has just carried his Goddess to a very special place where the Thunder and Lightning have created an orgasmic storm between her legs.

As the Goddess dismounts from the chariot, the male should thank her for sharing her pleasure with him, and ask if there is another way he might be of service to her. To honor your Goddess in this way, is to honor your relationship and the passion that has come into your home. The Goddess should honor the male partner for the assistance of getting her to a better place in this world.

The Goddess has a say in where she rides her chariot also. While she might decide to ride the chariot upon her bed, she also might want to venture to the couch or a chair. She might even want to ride her chariot in the bathtub during the royal bath. The beauty of it all is the Goddess can ride her chariot anyplace she wants—on a camping trip in a tent, on the dining room table after dinner, or even on the patio under the moonlight. Be adventurous, Goddess, and take your pleasure where it makes the most sense to you.

It is important for the male acting as the chariot to avoid ejaculating too soon and disrupting the Goddess's ride. It is also important for the male to prepare for the ride before it begins by adding extra pillows around the chariot, just in case the Goddess might fall from her chariot. Also prepare by having any items ready for the journey, such as condoms, lubrication, toys, etc.

CHAPTER 4: ORAL SEX POSITIONS FOR HER

GETTING ORAL SEX RIGHT
(TECHNIQUES FOR AMAZING ORAL SEX)

Oral sex on your female partner is an interesting-yet-foreign practice to many! While it can unlock the most amazing pleasure, it can also be mysterious, intimidating, and a huge learning process. Oral sex can be a truly amazing experience for her, but it can also be a huge pleasure for the giver as well. Many cultures believe that there is a great power that comes from the juices that flow from the vagina. The vagina is a passage to pleasure like no other, and for someone else to taste, lick, and ingest these juices is quite powerful; many believe that it can even extend your life. But how do we perform oral sex on our partner to the point of giving them enough pleasure to share their amazing juices with us? Well, rejoice—that is what this section is all about.

As I mentioned above, this can be a very mysterious journey for you as the giver of oral pleasure, so I have crafted an easy process to help you start the journey. One of the most interesting things in our world is the formation of crop circles in fields around the globe. Some believe they are man-made, and others believe that they are created by aliens from distant planets. Both theories have merit, but neither has any impact on our version of Delightful Crop circles. So forget about crop circles as you know them. The circular pattern of the crop circles is what we will be using to help guide you towards giving the most pleasure possible. The wonderful lady you are sharing this experience with will never look at crop circles the same again after experiencing this process. So start thinking in circles, as that is the example we are going to use as we unleash as much pleasure as we possibly can.

First things first: this is not meant to be something that happens fast, so if you are thinking you will do these Delightful Crop Circles as fast as you can, you are mistaken. Pleasure takes time, and the more build up to the climactic events, the more powerful they will be. Plus, if you do it right, you will be invited back more often—just think of your lady friend pushing your head down between her legs. That is the sign you are doing a fantastic job. Make sure to refer to the illustration as often as you need; most men are confused by the female anatomy, especially in the area we are going to be pleasuring.

Before we get started, let me also encourage you to be aware and pay attention during the process. Every amazing and beautiful woman is different, as are their sensations and sexual appetite. Watch for signs as you perform these Delightful Crop Circles on your partner; some signs will show what your partner really likes, while other signs will tell you it is time to move to another section. If you are lucky, you will have a partner who tells you when something feels really good. Otherwise you have to learn to interpret their body language, vocalizations, and even their breathing. Being aware and taking mental notes is a sure way to help improve each oral sexual connection.

Oral sex performed on women isn't just about your mouth, tongue, and lips. While those are super important, make sure to incorporate your hands, fingers, and nose, along with toys that can add to the experience. The important thing to focus on during this time is her pleasure. As the giver in this situation, it is your duty to use everything at your means to produce the desired effect. The upside to that is when you take the time and do it right, usually your partner will return the favor when it is your time to be the receiver.

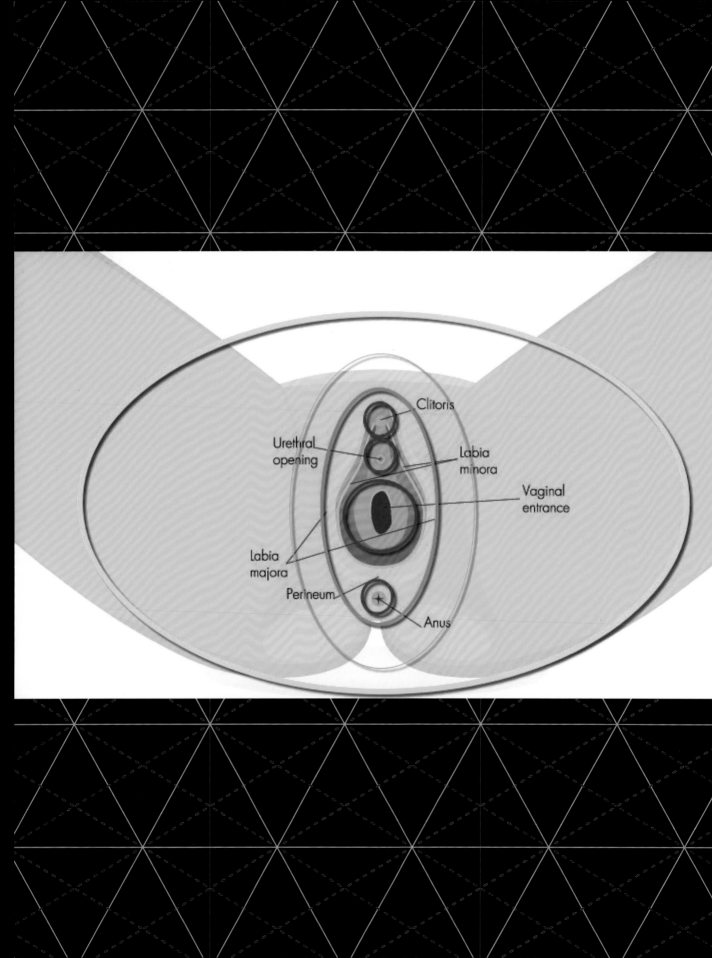

DELIGHTFUL CROP CIRCLES TECHNIQUE

Delightful Crop Circles have five levels we want to focus on. Those areas are: The Warm-Up Area, The Preheat Area, The Starting-to-Boil Area, The Boiling Area, and The Explosive Area. You need to pleasure these areas in order. However, you can always move back to an area to add excitement to the pleasure, but be cautious about jumping forward, as your partner might not be ready. Again, we don't want to rush; you need to spend adequate time in each area. Once you explore each area to the fullest, you will know your partner on a much more intimate and exciting level. Please refer to the illustration on the opposite page as often as needed to help give you a better understanding of the process.

THE WARM-UP AREA

This is where it all begins! You have made the commitment to giving your partner oral pleasure and the stage is yours. The Warm-Up Area, signified in yellow on the illustration, allows you to begin touching your partner without being too invasive from the start. That includes the legs and inner thighs, and you can even broaden the circle to include the entire leg, as you work your way up to the designated area in the illustration. Start by rubbing the area with your hands, careful not to go too far into the center. Be patient, my friends; we will get there, I promise. After your partner becomes accustomed to your touch, then move in, and use your nose, or rub your facial cheeks against her inner thighs. Now you can start to kiss, or maybe even lick, this area of the inner thighs, all the time paying attention to the signs that it is time to move to the next area. When your partner starts to open up her legs a little wider, that seems to be a pretty good sign to move to the next area.

THE PREHEAT AREA

Now we are ready to get cooking, but, like anything we bake, we are going to have to preheat the oven. The Preheat Area is shown on the illustration in orange. The areas included in this zone are the Mons Pubis (the area of fatty tissue that covers the pubic bone, or basically where the pubic hair would be located) and the Labia Majora, or the outer lips of the Labia. Start with touching with your fingers to get the blood flowing to these areas. Once they have been caressed, move your mouth towards them. Kissing, licking, and even sucking on these parts can be extremely arousing. These actions will start to heat up the rest of your partner's body in a major way. These areas can be part of your partner's erogenous spots, so pay attention to her reactions. At this point the vagina might be starting to lubricate itself, which is a good sign to move on, but avoid the temptation to move there quickly.

THE STARTING-TO-BOIL AREA

The areas in this oval, which is green in color on the illustration, include the Labia Minora (the inner lips of the labia), and the perineum (the area between the vagina opening and anus). At this point, you should start to feel and taste the juices your lover is producing. Start by sliding your fingers around the inner lips, and you should feel the wetness, or invitation, of the vagina. Hold off, however; I know this is difficult, but we want our partner to be screaming for this pleasure, and by taking our time, we are going to give her a more intense orgasm. Press your finger on the perineum and you should feel juices that have run out of the vagina. At this point, they might even be running down the entire perineum into the anus. Again, take your time. Hopefully by this time your partner is starting to squirm with each touch, anticipating the pleasure. Now move your mouth to these areas and begin to kiss, lick, and suck. Sucking on the inner lips can be extremely erotic. Take your time to explore, as you are getting into even more fascinating parts of your partner's body.

Remember, at any time you can go back to the previous areas to add more pleasure. If you have found a particular spot that seems to be a sensual button for your partner, then return to it while you are orally pleasuring another area. Keep your hands moving as often as you can, even if it is just to reach around and grab your partner's butt to pull them closer to your face. You can even move your hands up to the breasts and nipples to see how your partner responds to your mouth stimulating them, while you are fondling their breast or pinching their nipples. Just reading all this should be getting you a bit excited in itself.

THE BOILING AREA

Things should be moving along quite nicely. We're moving on to the inner purple circle on the diagram. Your partner's vagina should be wet with lubrication, and ready to enjoy some oral pleasure. If your partner does have some lubrication issues, as some people do, then make sure to have a good lube nearby so you don't lose the flow here. Now we are going to move to the tongue as the focal point of oral sex. Begin to lick at the opening of the vagina, slowly at first, and then it should become more welcoming to you to stick your tongue inside the vagina. Depending on the length of your tongue and makeup of your partner's body, you might even be able to hit the G-Spot with your tongue. Use your tongue to explore the vagina and, lucky you—you are starting to get to taste more of that golden elixir that comes from the vagina. With your tongue inside your partner exploring, you can use your fingers around the opening of the vagina to increase the pleasure. It is possible that your partner might orgasm at this point. However, many women don't orgasm in this manner. But don't worry, we have the Explosive Zone still yet to go.

Your partner should be working into a frenzy. I want you to think about your actions now as a circus. Keep as much action going in as many different rings, (or circles in our case), as you can. Keep your mouth, tongue, and lips moving around your partner's genital area, and also keep those hands as part of the experience. If you want to orally pleasure another part of your partner's body, you might want to slide a finger or two into her vagina while you kiss another part of her body. Feel free to experiment at this point and see what works.

THE EXPLOSIVE AREA

Okay, it is time for blast off, the best efforts to give your partner the oral orgasm of a lifetime. The explosive zone has three main areas of focus: the Clitoris, Urethral Opening, and the Anus. All three of these areas, shown with the blue circles on the diagram, can be hot spots to bring about orgasms. The Clitoris is usually the most sensitive of the three. Be prepared in advance: the Clitoris can usually only stand so much pleasure, but your partner will tell you or push you away when you hit that point, so it will be obvious. Just understand that most of the time, it will happen. The Urethral Opening is where urine comes out of the female, and some claim it is also the area that ejaculate comes out of the woman, so if you have seen any video of squirters, you might want to be prepared for this, because if it happens it can be a gusher. Now the Anus is an area some people are afraid to approach, but it is also an area that is full of nerve endings that can push your partner over the edge. Let's focus on these areas one at a time.

Most people know about the magical ability of the clitoris to bring about orgasm. But there are so many techniques to pleasuring it orally. First there is the circle, where you take your tongue and circle the clitoris. You partner might like you to do this fast, or they might like it slow, so test it out to see for yourself. The flick is another wonderful way to get the clitoris aroused. The flick is just using your tongue to flick the clitoris back and forth. Depending on your lover, the hood or skin that covers the clitoris can also be used for pleasure. Pushing with a little more pressure on the hood of the clitoris can really get a reaction from the clitoris underneath. Another favorite is sucking the clitoris; this takes some practice, but, once mastered, allows you to use the above techniques to a higher degree. Once you locate the clitoris on your partner, you gently suck on it like you would a straw, bringing it more out into the open for the other pleasures. Don't be afraid to use your fingers to make it easier to reach the clitoris, and you can even move back and forth using your fingers and mouth to get a different experience. Speed is another thing to consider, and it will differ for each woman. Some like it slow, and some might like it fast. You will have to pay attention to your partner; maybe they will like a mixture of speeds. The clitoris is one of the most enjoyable things to play with on a woman's body, and she will most likely be just as excited as you are about it.

The Urethral Opening is seldom spoken about in oral pleasure, and maybe because it is the place where urine exits the body. The urethral opening is located just down from the Clitoris and before the opening of the vagina. It is thought to be the location of expulsion of the ejaculate. It you are lucky enough to experience this, you would be amazed at the amount of fluid that comes from female ejaculation. It seems that not all women are capable of this ability, but you never know when the first time might happen. However, using your tongue to stimulate this area is very pleasurable for many women.

There are so many people afraid to approach the anus, especially in oral pleasure. However, it can be a huge benefit to your partner and power their orgasm. First, let's talk about rimming. Rimming is running your tongue around the rim of your partner's anus. This stimulates all the nerves endings around the anus, and will really add a level of excitement to all the other things going on. Now you can also perform Anilingus on your partner, which involves rimming, as well as inserting the tongue into the anus. That can be extremely exciting to your partner. Please remember that while hygiene is always important, it is extremely important with anal play.

IN SUMMARY

Delightful Crop Circles are a wonderful experience for your female partner. But it is also a wonderful experience for you, too. The connection and sharing of the experience is something that many wish and hope to achieve. I encourage everyone to think about circles the entire time they are performing these activities. There is something sexy about circles, and something mystical about them, also. So, when are you are orally pleasuring any part of your partner, keep in mind the power of the circle and move around the body in a circular motion. It is a constant flow of pleasure moving around the entire body.

There are so many variations to add to Delightful Crop Circles. Adding the sensations of toys is a great way to increase the experience. Even some arm and leg restraints could make the experience more pleasurable. There are endless ways to bring new and exciting pleasure to the area. The best part is that it can be a little different each and every time you perform oral sex and Delightful Crop Circles on your partner. Things as simple as moving from the bed to a chair or the dining room table can change the experience. The best part for the ladies is that they get to lay back and let someone else drive them on the road of pleasure, stopping from spot to spot to lay down a Delightful Crop Circle.

"Oral Sex is the language of love that never needs a translator."

ORAL SEX TONGUE EXERCISES FOR MEN & WOMEN

Your tongue is a muscle; did you know that? If not, you do now. This muscle is super important for having amazing sexual experiences. Your tongue muscle is important for tasting, licking, swallowing, and articulating speech, all of which are important to our sex life. This is why the exercises below are so important to practice on a daily basis. Keeping your tongue in shape will take your sexual encounters into a new dimension. The best part is that you can do your tongue exercises anywhere and almost at any time. You might not want to do all of them in your next work meeting, though, if you want to keep your job.

Before we get started with the exercises, let's talk a bit about how these exercises are going to improve your relationship. First of all, communication in any relationship is the key, and with a stronger tongue you are better able to articulate words, so these exercises are improving communication. Now, the exercises won't keep you from saying stupid things, but you will be able to say them more clearly and more articulately.

Licking with your tongue will become a very special experience once you start performing these exercises on a regular basis. If I really need to explain why licking is important in your sexual endeavors, we need to start completely over. Whether you swallow or not is your choice, but these exercises will make you the master at it, if you so desire. The flavors of love will also be better as you strengthen your tongue, allowing you a wider range of the taste sensations that come along with sex. Lastly, your kissing will become that of legend, putting you right up there with Casanova and Don Juan.

Each exercise I will teach you, I have done many times over in my life, and continue to do to this day. Your tongue can never get too strong. Don't worry about it getting too big to fit in your mouth; nature will not allow that to happen, unless you get it stung by some flying insect. Some of these exercises might be difficult to do, or even impossible to do at first, but, just like any other exercise program, the more diligently you stay at them, the better the results will be. Soon you will be the most amazing tongue master ever, and your lover will really appreciate it. Now, as with any exercise program, please consult your physician before putting any stress on any muscle. And please record it when you ask your doctor if your tongue is healthy enough for sexual exercises.

Okay, on to the exercises. The first thing we need to do is warm that amazing muscle in your mouth up. So take a few minutes to roll your tongue around the inside of your mouth. Rub it around the roof of your mouth, then move it around your mouth by placing the tip of your tongue on the front side of your teeth, and move it around to touch all your teeth, top and bottom. Do this about ten times on the upper and lower teeth, then switch and do the inside side your teeth, again doing ten reps on the upper and lower sets of teeth. For the last part of the warm up, take your tongue and just stick it out like a bratty little kid would. Do this ten times and you might already be starting to feel some fatigue in your jaws. This is normal, and as you do these exercises more and more, your stamina will get better and better, which will be great for when you have those long lovemaking sessions with your partner.

Next, we are going to do what I call tongue yoga! This is moving the tongue in slow and controlled movements, allowing the tongue to stretch. You will see improvement in this as you go along, but don't be disappointed at first. These moves are not designed to be done fast, so don't try to get them done as quickly as possible. First, stick your tongue out in front of you as far as it will go, doing this ten times. Next, let your tongue slide down the front of your chin and see how far it will go. Do this in the mirror, so you can see the improvement as it starts to happen. Push your tongue a little to see how far you can stretch it down your chin. Do this for ten reps. Next, see if you can touch the tip of your tongue to the tip of your nose for ten reps. For the last section of tongue yoga, stick your tongue out to the side of your mouth as if you are trying to touch your cheeks. Do each side here for ten reps. Your tongue is now in a more peaceful place after this tongue yoga!

Now we are moving on to the speed area of our tongue exercises. Let's start by sticking our tongue out and moving it up and down as fast as we can. Let it flap against your upper and lower lips. See how long you can do this; try to do it for at least ten seconds. Next, do the same, except moving your tongue from side to side as fast as you can. For the last part of our speed section, rub your tongue around the outer part of your lips, making a circle around your both your upper and lower lips. Try to keep your tongue connected at all times with your lips. Do ten seconds in one direction, and then try to switch directions. This is a lot more difficult than it sounds. The speed your tongue moves can be the driving force in pushing your partner to orgasm.

It is now time to sculpt your tongue. Basically, we are going to see how many different shapes you can move your tongue into. Start out by sticking your tongue out and keeping it pointed, making sure your tongue stays narrow. Do that for ten reps, then switch it up and see how wide you can make your tongue. See if you can make your tongue wide enough to touch both sides of your mouth as you stick your tongue out. If you are watching in the mirror, you will see how much different your tongue looks now when compared to when you were making it narrow. Now think about how different that will feel when you are placing it on your partner. Next, let's try to roll your tongue up, making it look like a straw. Some of you will be able to do this easily, and for others this will be challenging. See if there are any other shapes you can make with your tongue. Now you have completed three sections of tongue exercises.

I feel compelled to share with you some advanced exercise to help you with your tongue development. The first being to get an individual container of ice cream and eat it without the use of a spoon. At first, it will be easy, but as you get further down in the container it will stretch the limits of your tongue. Make sure to take notice of the different shapes your tongue gets into while you are doing this. Now, let's put some resistance on your tongue. Take your index and middle finger, and place them on top of your tongue, and then, with your tongue, try to push up on those fingers. This really works the back part of your tongue.

Now, my last little tip here is my secret weapon to help you pleasure your partner. What you do is stick the tip of your index finger in your mouth, then suck on your index finger and, while you are sucking on your finger, take your tongue and either roll it around the tip of your finger, or flick your finger with your tongue in an up and down motion or side to side. This little tip will help create an amazing sensation for your partner, whether you replace the index finger with the tip of your male partner's penis, or your female partner's clitoris.

Well, there you have it, the workout for your tongue that will create some amazing pleasure and will help you become an oral sex god or goddess.

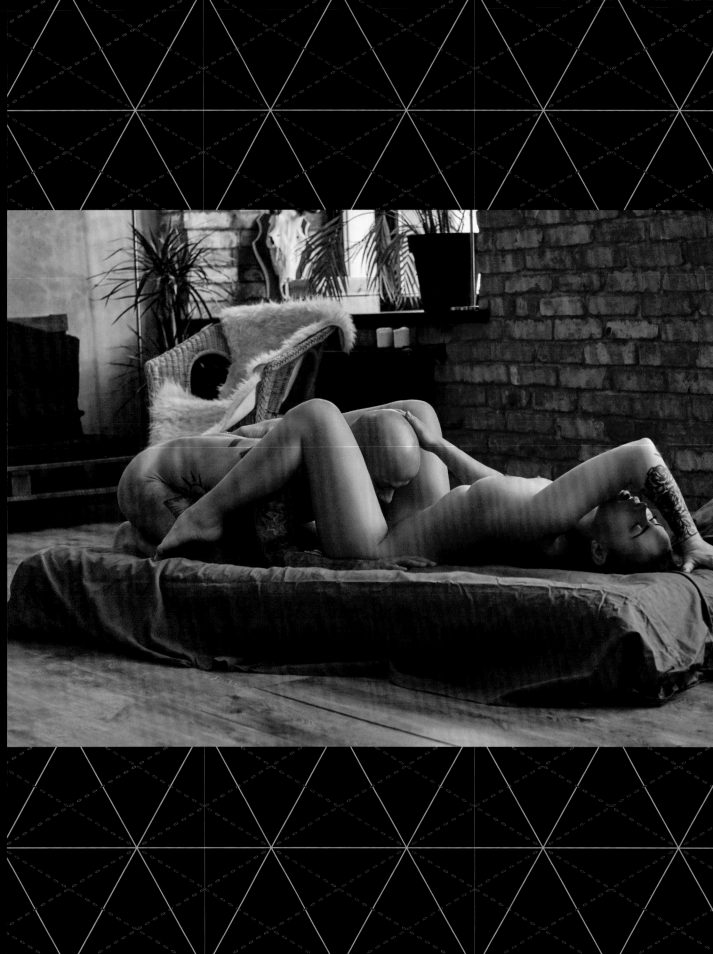

SPREAD EAGLE

This classic oral sex position is a tried-and-true standard for many couples. Although it lacks the "exotic" factor, it's a favorite among women because they can simply lie back, relax, and enjoy the pleasure!

HOW TO DO IT

This is the "Missionary" of oral sex positions for her. It's the most common oral sex position for women, and it's actually a favorite, simply because the female partner has the ability to relax and focus on the pleasurable sensations she's receiving. For many women, relaxation and focus are critical components to achieving orgasm! The female partner lies on her back with her legs spread, and her male partner situates himself in between her legs, so that he can give her oral sex. It's simple, but very, very effective!

WHERE TO DO IT

While this position can be done just about anywhere, the comfort of a soft bed will help her relax and enjoy herself more.

PROPS YOU'LL NEED

Adding a pillow under her lower back will tilt her pelvis up and give her partner more access to her vulva.

DIFFICULTY LEVEL ★☆☆☆☆

HER O-METER ★★★★★

Women love the Spread-Eagle oral sex position because they're able to lie back, relax, and enjoy everything. They only have to focus on what feels good, which can be exactly what a woman needs to reach orgasm.

HIS O-METER ★☆☆☆☆

This is probably the least favorite oral sex position among men, simply because it can make for some serious neck cramps! It's not easy getting the angle right when licking, and the neck can bend in an odd way. Some men may not be able to keep this position up long enough to actually bring their lovers to orgasm. He also can't reach down and stimulate himself very well.

MAKE IT HOTTER...

Guys, slip a lubed finger inside her vagina, and gently massage her G-spot, while you lick her clitoris (after she's warmed up and turned on, of course!). This will increase her chances of orgasm, and if you do it well enough, you may even get her to squirt!

Bottoms Up

The Bottoms-Up sex position is an oral sex position for her that puts her in an extremely vulnerable, yet naughty and erotic, pose! It's only for the adventurous!

HOW TO DO IT

The female partner lies on her back, grasps her hips, and raises her buttocks in the air, letting her legs fall back towards her head. The male partner rests his weight on his knees, and helps hold her hips for stability as he goes down on her from above. What makes the Bottoms-Up sex position so incredibly naughty is that it completely exposes both her vulva and anal areas for him to stimulate with his mouth as he pleases. This is an oral sex position that should definitely only be performed by couples who are extremely comfortable with each other, and women who are exceptionally self-confident!

If she is not able to get into this position, have her pull her knees to her chest and spread her legs as far as comfortable.

WHERE TO DO IT

The bed is the best place for the Bottoms-Up sex position simply because the female partner is in such an awkward position, that she'll take any bit of comfort she can get. This can also be done on the sofa, but the floor is going to be a little too firm for her to truly be comfortable there for any length of time.

PROPS YOU'LL NEED

She may want a pillow for her neck and upper shoulders. A Liberator Wedge is a great way for her to easily stay in position without getting too tired from holding herself up.

DIFFICULTY LEVEL ★★★★☆

HER O-METER ★★★★☆

If she's super adventurous and kinky, she will absolutely love the Bottoms-Up sex position. She'll love feeling spread out and vulnerable to her partner! If she's not very flexible, however, this position may be fairly uncomfortable for her. It's definitely one she'll want to try, though, if she's comfortable with her partner.

HIS O-METER ★☆☆☆☆

He will enjoy the Bottoms Up sex position if he really digs giving oral sex, or even if he likes giving anilingus. This sex position doesn't force him to crane his neck in any way, making it one of the more comfortable oral sex positions for him.

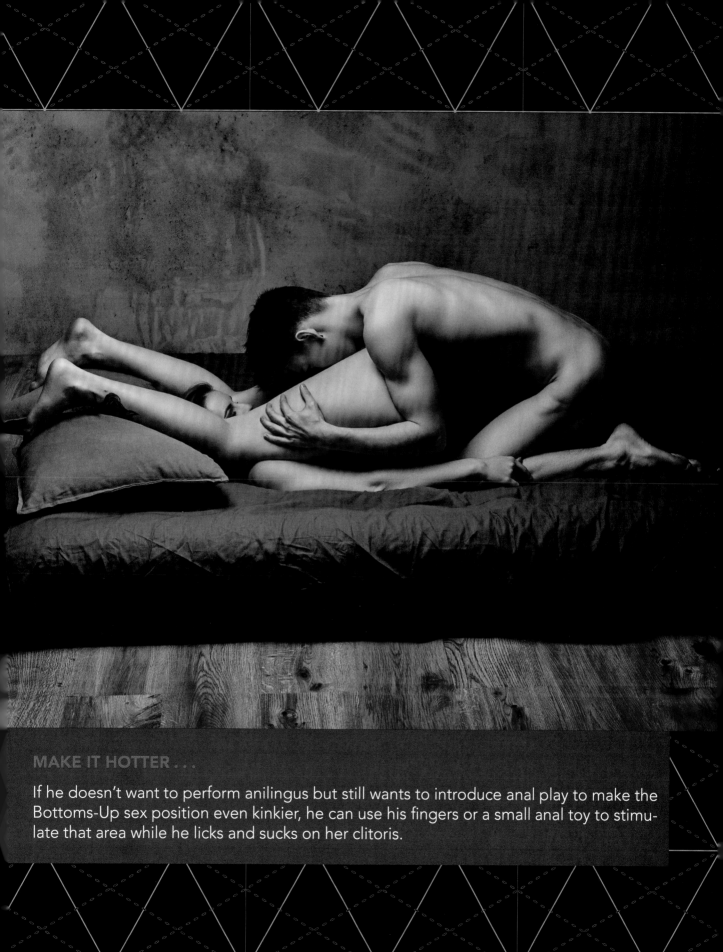

MAKE IT HOTTER . . .

If he doesn't want to perform anilingus but still wants to introduce anal play to make the Bottoms-Up sex position even kinkier, he can use his fingers or a small anal toy to stimulate that area while he licks and sucks on her clitoris.

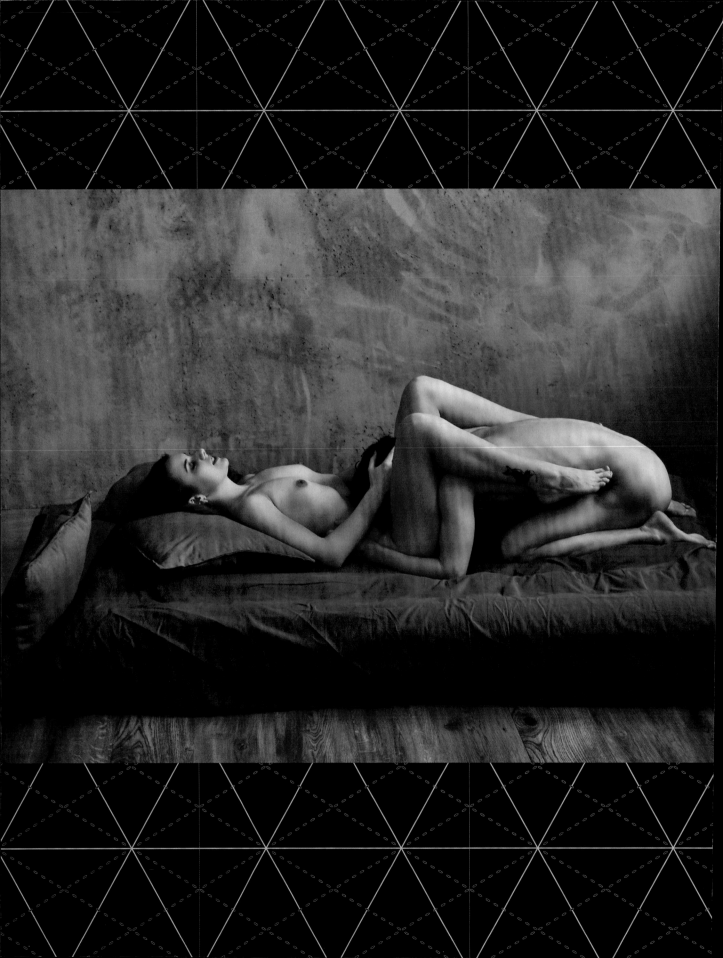

EAR WARMER

The Ear-Warmer sex position is a simple variation of the Spread Eagle (see page 87), where she has more control and may be more comfortable than with her legs spread.

HOW TO DO IT

The female partner lies back and spreads her legs long enough for her partner to lie on his stomach and place his head in between her legs to give her oral sex. Instead of keeping her legs spread like with the Spread-Eagle sex position, though, she closes her legs somewhat, resting her inner thighs on either side of her lover's head. This gives her more control during cunnilingus, and many women may be more comfortable with their hips at this angle.

WHERE TO DO IT

The bed is a super comfortable and familiar area to perform this position, but it can also be done on the edge of the bed (with her partner resting his knees on the floor), or on a sofa.

PROPS YOU'LL NEED

Add a pillow for her head, and possibly under her lower back to place her hips at an angle that makes oral sex easier for him to give.

DIFFICULTY LEVEL ★☆☆☆☆

HER O-METER ★★★★

With increased control and comfort, she can really lie back and relax in the Ear-Warmer sex position. She loves receiving oral sex, and in this position he's totally and completely focusing on her pleasure.

HIS O-METER ★☆☆☆☆

The Ear-Warmer sex position may not be his favorite if he wants to have more freedom for head movement. He may feel a little confined with her legs pressed up against his head.

MAKE IT HOTTER . . .

He can easily use one of his hands to stimulate her G-spot while he's licking her clitoris, which will bring her to orgasm even faster.

FACE STRADDLE

The Face Straddle is an excellent oral sex position to use when the female partner wants to feel in control of oral sex, and the male partner wants to feel a little submissive. It also gives him a great view of her body as she writhes in pleasure!

HOW TO DO IT

Face Straddle is an oral sex position for her, and it can be a lot of fun if both partners are very comfortable with each other. Some women may not like the idea of straddling their partner's face, while some men won't like the fact that they have limited head and neck movement—especially if she starts getting into it and grinding her pelvis into his face. However, for some couples, this move is really hot! The male partner assumes a lying position and the female partner lowers her genitals over his face, straddling his head with each leg on one side. There are a couple different ways to do this, but both require her to rest her weight on her knees. She can lean back and rest the remainder of her weight on her hands, or she can lean forward and get on all fours. Either way, this provides her lover with complete access to her genitals.

WHERE TO DO IT

Try the sofa, bed, floor, or back seat of the car—anywhere with enough space to lie down.

PROPS YOU'LL NEED

A pillow for his neck is a definite must!

DIFFICULTY LEVEL ★☆☆☆☆

HER O-METER ★★★★☆

This is an excellent oral sex position for her because she feels more in control here. She can move her pelvis to guide her clitoris to where she wants it to be, and she can rock and move in a way that gets her closer to orgasm. She's not relying only on him to get her there.

HIS O-METER ★★★☆☆

Many men enjoy this position, because they feel a little submissive here. Also, if a man isn't that confident at oral sex, he may feel better that she can maneuver herself, so that she gets more pleasure, rather than relying only on him and his tongue movements to get her off.

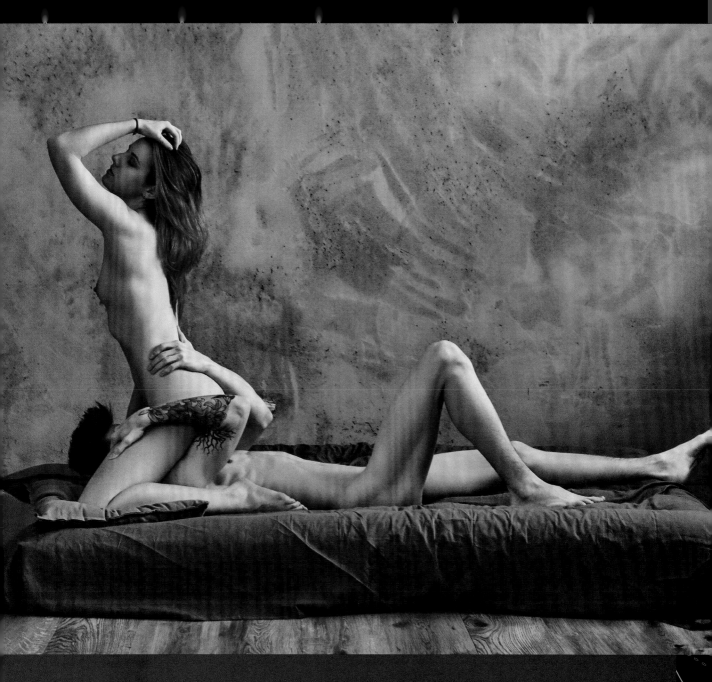

MAKE IT HOTTER . . .

Guys, reach down and masturbate while you're giving her oral sex. She won't necessarily be able to look behind her to see what you're doing, but the idea that you love eating her out so much that you can't help but touch yourself is extremely erotic for her, especially considering that many women feel that guys think oral sex is a chore.

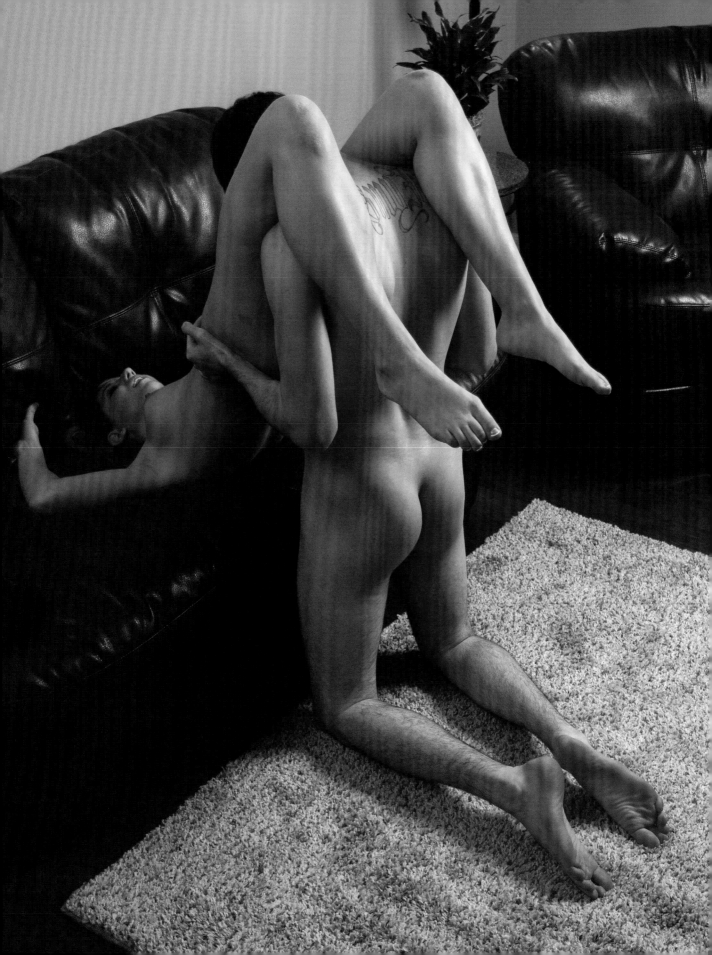

FEEDBAG

The Feedbag sex position is an interesting oral sex position that can be a little challenging for her, but is very rewarding once it is accomplished.

HOW TO DO IT

The female partner lies on the sofa with her rear at the edge of it and her legs and feet hanging off. Her partner then kneels in front of her, lifts her buttocks with his hands, and places her legs over his shoulders. It's a tight fit for his head to get in between her legs, but it can be a lot of fun once you get into this position.

WHERE TO DO IT

The sofa is the best place for the Feedbag sex position.

PROPS YOU'LL NEED

She may want a small pillow for her neck and upper shoulders, and he'll appreciate a pillow, blanket, or towel for his knees to rest on instead of the floor.

DIFFICULTY LEVEL ★★★★☆

HER O-METER ★★★☆☆

The Feedbag probably isn't going to be her favorite position for oral sex, but hey, she's getting it, so it's all good, right? Her legs aren't spread very wide at all here, so her lover has limited access to the nerves on her inner labia and even parts of her clitoris. She's also in a bit of an awkward position; however, the blood rushing to her head can intensify her orgasm if he can get her there.

HIS O-METER ★☆☆☆☆

If he really likes being enveloped by his lover's vulva and legs, he's going to love the Feedbag sex position, but he'll likely enjoy other oral sex positions more if he wants more control or freedom of movement.

MAKE IT HOTTER . . .

He can easily reach forward and caress her thighs and belly, as well as stimulating her breasts and nipples with his hands!

Leg Up

This hot oral sex position for her is simple for both partners. The Leg Up gives him full access to her, while making it easy for her to watch.

HOW TO DO IT

The female partner stands next to a chair, sofa, low table, or other surface, and raises one leg at a ninety-degree angle, so she can rest her foot on the surface and spread her legs. Her partner sits on the floor cross-legged beneath her, with his head positioned in between her legs. He can grasp her hips or play with her breasts while he goes down on her in the Leg-Up sex position.

WHERE TO DO IT

You can do the Leg-Up sex position anywhere you can put one foot up!

PROPS YOU'LL NEED

A chair, sofa, low table, or bed that is the proper height for her to rest her foot on so that she is comfortable. He may also want a pillow, small blanket, or a towel to sit on, as he will be sitting on the floor.

DIFFICULTY LEVEL ★☆☆☆☆

HER O-METER ★★★★☆

What she loves about the Leg-Up sex position is that she's not only comfortable, but spread open wide enough for him to access her most sensitive parts. She can watch the action here, which is not always the case in other oral sex positions. This is an entirely new way for her to experience oral sex! The one downside is that it may be difficult to reach orgasm from the standing position.

HIS O-METER ★★★☆☆

He's comfortable in the Leg-Up sex position too, and loves being able to grasp her buttocks, or raise his hands up and fondle her breasts, while he goes down on her.

MAKE IT HOTTER . . .

Her hands are fairly unoccupied in the Leg-Up sex position, so she can use them to either stimulate her own nipples or reach down and spread her labia wide for him. The latter will take the Leg-Up sex position up a few notches and make it way hotter than it already is!

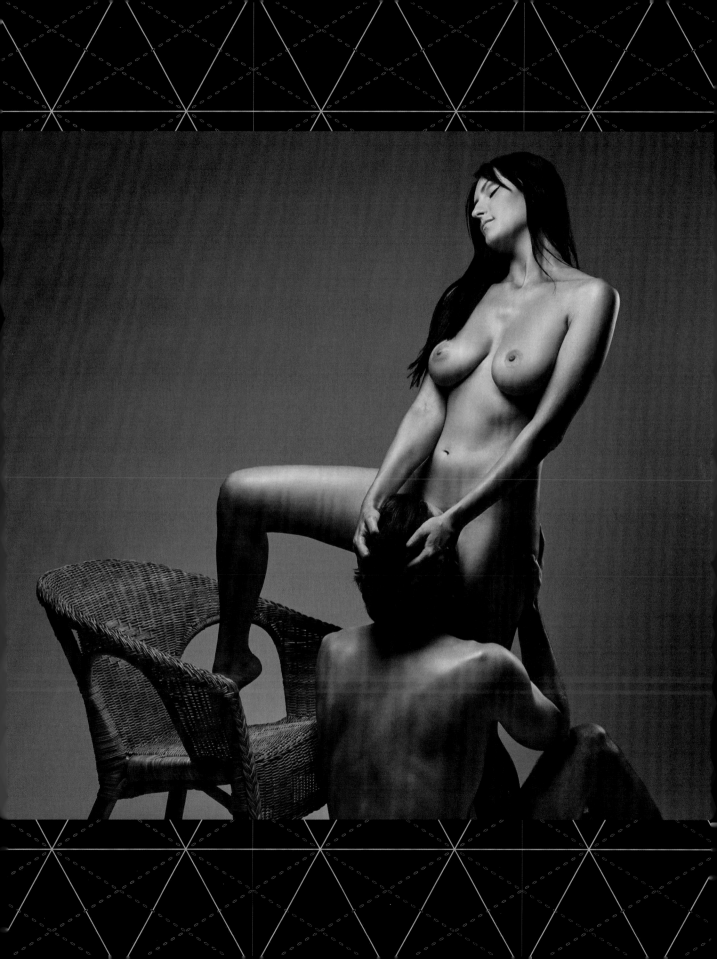

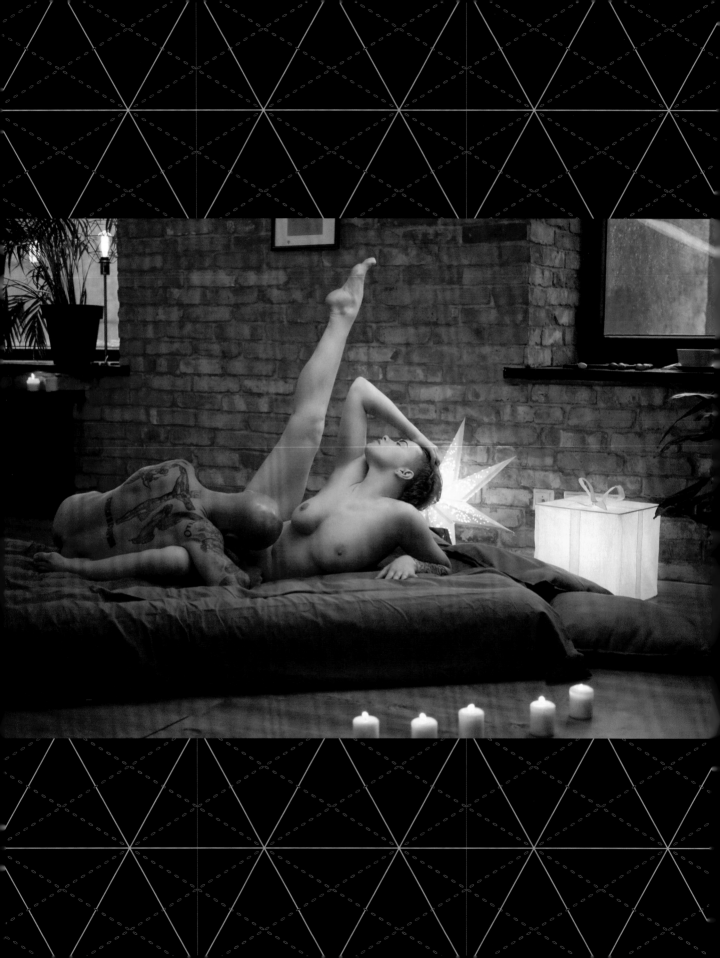

LICKING THE FLAGPOLE

The Licking-the-Flagpole sex position is a comfortable oral sex position for both her and him, which leaves her spread wide open for the ultimate pleasure.

HOW TO DO IT

The Licking-the-Flagpole sex position is easy to get into. The female partner simply lies on her side on the bed, with her bottom leg bent at the knee to give her stability. She then lifts her top leg high in the air, placing her hand on her thigh to help hold it up. The male partner then lies on his side perpendicular to her, and rests his head on her bottom thigh while he goes down on her.

WHERE TO DO IT

This is OK on a floor or other wide-open space, but both partners will appreciate the comfort of the bed with surrounding pillows.

PROPS YOU'LL NEED

Use pillows as needed for extra support.

DIFFICULTY LEVEL ★☆☆☆☆

HER O-METER ★★★★☆

She loves being spread out for him, because this position gives him access to every nerve in her clitoris and labia. The only caveat is that if she's not very flexible or athletic, she may have trouble stretching her leg that high, and keeping it there for a significant period of time. It's fine to put a slight bend in the knee of the top leg to make it more comfortable.

HIS O-METER ★☆☆☆☆

He enjoys the comfort of this position, and it's very easy on the neck. Since her inner thigh is supporting his head, he's quite comfortable and relaxed while giving her oral sex.

MAKE IT HOTTER . . .

If she enjoys anal play, Licking the Flagpole is perfect for him to give her simultaneous oral sex and anal stimulation with his hands. It's a great way to make this sex position even naughtier than it already is!

REVERSE FACE STRADDLE

One of the "kinkier" oral sex positions for her, the Reverse Face Straddle is not for the shy or timid woman. Because it involves her partner's face and nose so close to her backdoor, she needs to be super comfortable with her partner. But it's an excellent position for couples who enjoy anal play!

HOW TO DO IT

This is an oral sex position for her that requires quite a bit of confidence on her part, and both partners definitely need to be comfortable with each other. A sexy shower beforehand is also a must! As with the forward-facing version of this oral sex position, the male partner lies on a bed, sofa, or the floor (any flat surface will do), and the female partner straddles his face, with one leg on either side of his head, resting her weight on her knees. The difference with this position is that she's facing his feet, as in the Reverse-Cowgirl sex position. He is able to perform oral sex on her from behind, and this is actually an excellent oral sex position for couples who enjoy anilingus. Because her rear is right in his face, she's clean, and trimmed, or shaved. He's going to feel better about it too!

WHERE TO DO IT

The Reverse Straddle can be done on the sofa, back seat of the car, floor, or any flat surface.

PROPS YOU'LL NEED

Use a pillow or rolled-up towel to support the male partner's neck.

DIFFICULTY LEVEL ★★★☆☆

HER O-METER ★★★☆☆

This is an oral sex position that really kinky women enjoy! Because she's so exposed to him, she's definitely got to have some confidence, and both partners need to be comfortable with each other. If she's shy or doesn't feel clean down there, this position could really backfire. But for women who want oral sex that is a little naughty, this position is a great one to use!

HIS O-METER ★★★☆☆

Men who like to be dominated (and men who like things a little kinky, or have a butt fetish) will really enjoy this oral sex position. Guys, you can up the pleasure factor for yourself by reaching down and masturbating while you're giving her oral sex. Since she's facing your feet, she'll be able to see you touch yourself, and it will turn her on like you wouldn't believe!

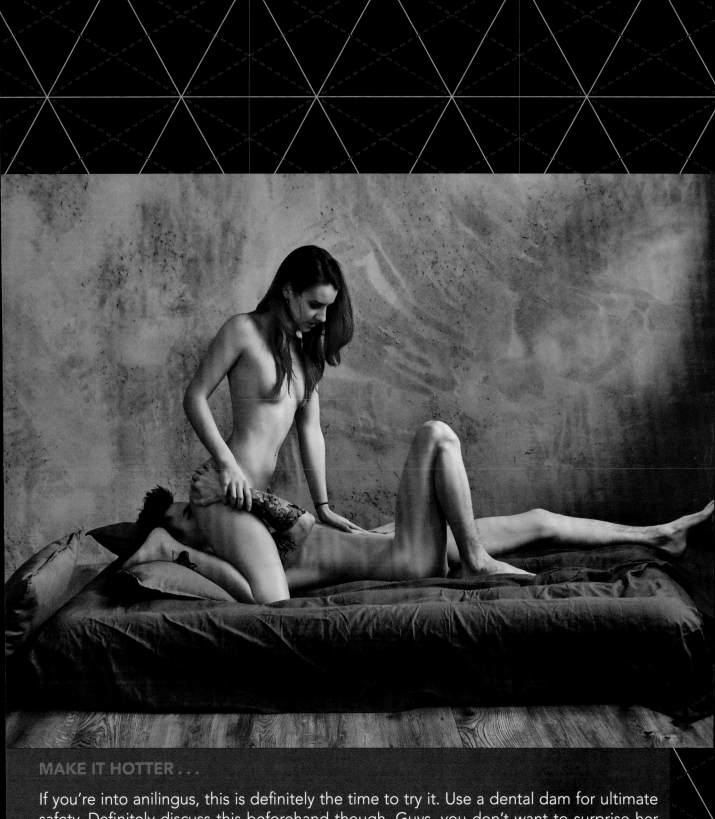

MAKE IT HOTTER . . .

If you're into anilingus, this is definitely the time to try it. Use a dental dam for ultimate safety. Definitely discuss this beforehand though. Guys, you don't want to surprise her with a tongue up her bum if she hasn't agreed to it first!

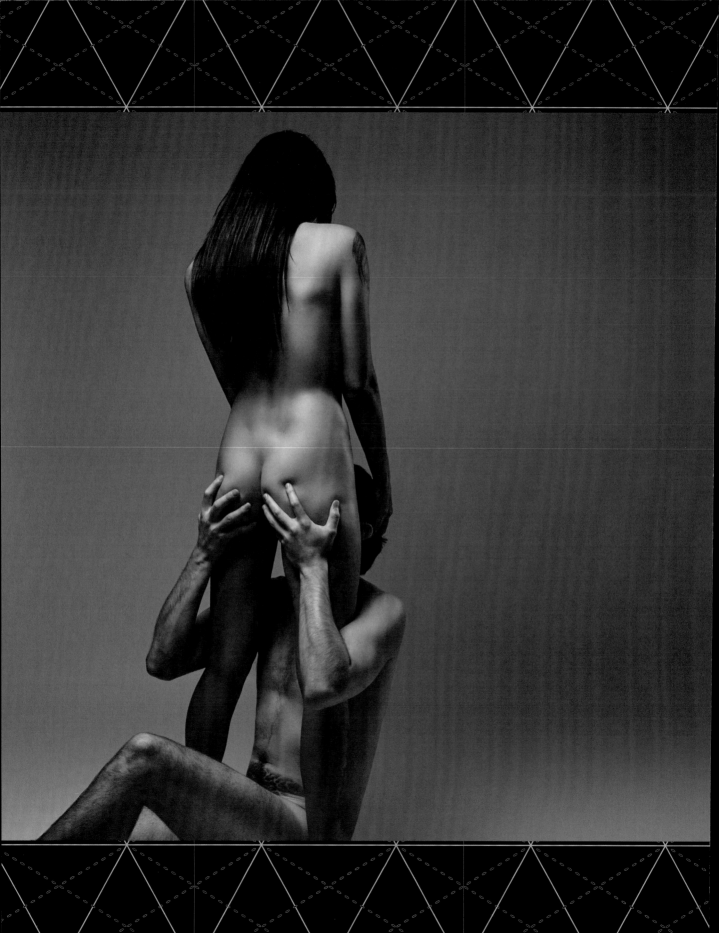

STANDING FACE STRADDLE

The Standing-Face-Straddle sex position is a fun and easy oral sex position for her that puts her in control. He likes it almost as much as she does!

HOW TO DO IT

The male partner sits on the floor with his legs crossed, and his partner stands above him, lowering her groin onto his face. He holds onto her hips for more stability, and she can use her hands to caress her own breasts and stimulate her nipples. It's quick and easy, but it's a very satisfying oral sex position for her.

WHERE TO DO IT

The Standing-Face-Straddle sex position is awesome for an oral sex quickie, because it can be done pretty much anywhere you have enough space. He doesn't have to get undressed, and all she really has to do is drop her drawers!

PROPS YOU'LL NEED

None.

DIFFICULTY LEVEL ★☆☆☆☆

HER O-METER ★★★★★

She loves being in control in the Standing-Face-Straddle sex position, especially considering that she can easily grind against his face to achieve an intense orgasm.

HIS O-METER ★☆☆☆☆

Submissive guys will like the Standing-Face-Straddle sex position; however, guys who like to be in control may not enjoy it as much. If she starts grinding too hard, it can become a bit uncomfortable. Communicate with your partner non-verbally if she starts to get a little too aggressive, or you feel like you're suffocating!

MAKE IT HOTTER . . .

He can use his fingers to stimulate her G-spot, while she can control the tempo and depth of her thrusting. It's the best of both worlds. A good G-spot vibrator is an incredible addition to this position!

Under the Hood (For Her)

The Under-the-Hood oral sex position is one that gives her partner full access to her nether region, and makes her feel exceptionally exposed.

HOW TO DO IT

The female partner lies on her back, and brings her legs and knees as close to her chest as possible. Typically, her legs are stretched out, but if this is difficult for her to do, a slight bend in the knee is OK. She can hold the backs of her thighs to help support her legs. The male partner then kneels to give his partner oral sex.

WHERE TO DO IT

A wide space like the bed or floor is best for the Under the Hood, but the bed is of course going to be much more comfortable.

PROPS YOU'LL NEED

She will want a pillow under her head, and he'll want one under his knees, if he's on the floor. A rolled-up blanket or towel will also work.

DIFFICULTY LEVEL ★☆☆☆☆

HER O-METER ★★★★☆

If she's not comfortable with her anal area being exposed, she's not going to like this sex position very much. However, for women who are totally comfortable with themselves, this one is a must try! It's totally hot!

HIS O-METER ★☆☆☆☆

He likes the Under-the-Hood oral sex position because it gives her the opportunity to feel vulnerable and him the opportunity to be in complete control.

MAKE IT HOTTER . . .

For a bondage twist, restrain her hands with ties and hold her legs in the fully-raised position, while giving her pleasure.

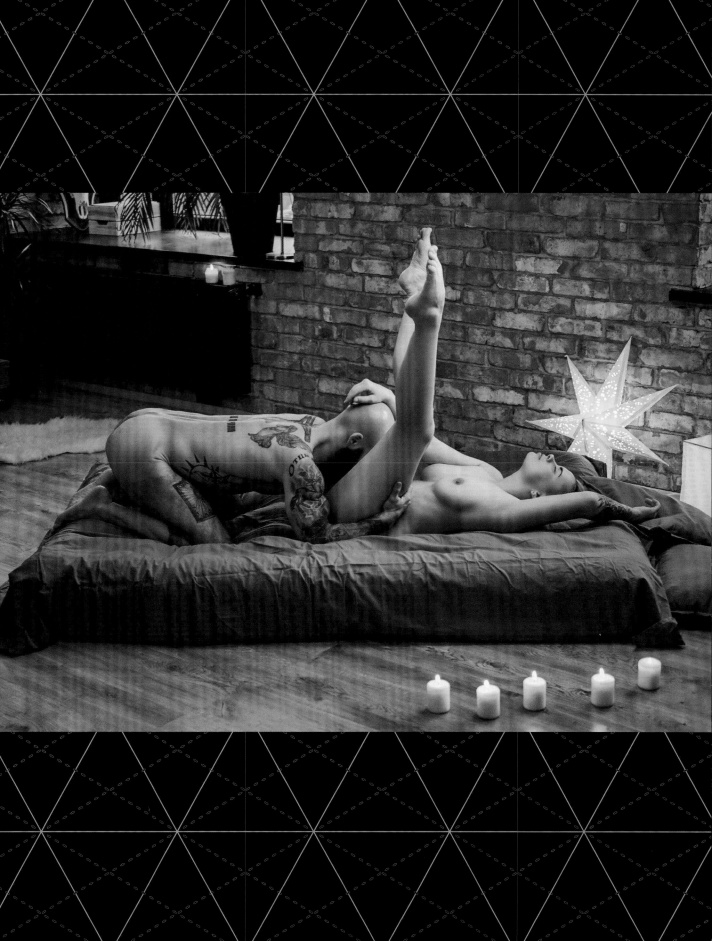

SEXY CHALLENGE:

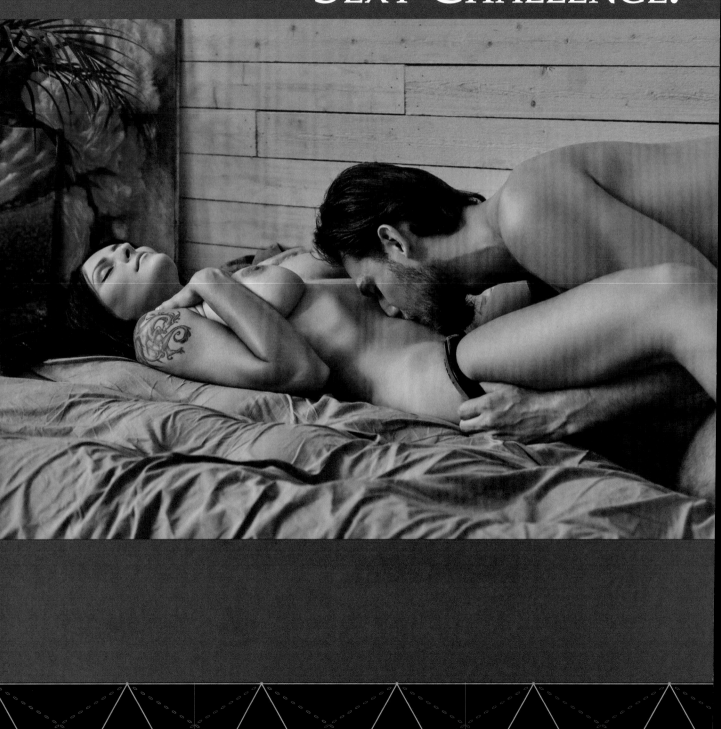

THE FEAST

Have you ever looked at an anatomy book? Women have an amazing amount of parts to make oral sex fun and exciting. While most males might look at this as an overwhelming task, if you look at it as an adventure, you will have a lot more fun performing oral sex on your female partner. When you think of performing oral sex on your female partner, you should approach it as a feast. A feast is defined as a large amount of food in celebration, and that definition works perfectly here because the female body offers a plethora of choices, and this is an amazing celebration of pleasure.

The important thing to remember is that you need to try a little bit of everything when you are having a Feast of Oral Sex with your female partner. Don't focus in only one area, or you will miss the entire experience of the feast. Plus, this is a celebration for the female you are preparing to feast upon, and will also be a celebration for the male involved. The feast should be laid before you for you to make your choices, so I would suggest trying the positions from this chapter like the Spread Eagle, Bottoms Up, Ear Warmer, or Under the Hood. These positions allow the male partner the easiest access to choose which parts of his partner's body he will be feasting upon. (See page 75 for The Delightful Crop Circles Technique)

Our feast will begin with the appetizer, to get warmed up. The appetizer is a combination of using your hands, mouth, and tongue to pleasure your female partner so that she is ready to offer up the main course. During the appetizer, focus on touching, kissing, and licking the following areas: Mons Pubis (this is the area usually covered by pubic hair), the Labia Majora, or the Outer Lips of the Vagina, the inner thighs, and buttocks. While these are not normally the most sensitive areas on a woman, they are great place to start sending signals to the other more sensitive areas.

Begin by touching, licking, and kissing the inner thighs, taking the time to see and feel when you might hit a sensitive spot. Use your hands to caress these areas, adding even more sensation to the experience. Slip your hands under your partner's buttocks to massage them or grip them, as you continue to run your mouth and tongue around the aforementioned areas. Watch for signs that your partner is ready for you to move to the next course of the feast. Take your time, however; many men tend to move too quickly to the next areas of the feast. The more time you spend enjoying each course of the feast, the more you will be rewarded and appreciated later.

Moving on to the second course of the feast, we start to heat things up even more, focusing on the more sensitive parts to enhance the enjoyment of your female partner. The areas we want to focus on during this course are the Labia Minora (inner lips), the vagina opening, and the perineum. Now, even though we are moving to the next level of pleasure, don't abandon the areas we have already been stimulating. Instead, just keep adding to the pleasure. Continue to focus on the areas mentioned in the appetizer, but include these new areas as well.

As you focus your attention on the second course, watch for signs that things are progressing nicely. Your female partner might start providing some guidance for you with her body language, so pay attention. Take some time to lick gently across the opening of the vagina. If things are going as expected, you will start to see and feel the opening becoming moist with lubrication. This is a very good sign that you are almost ready to move on to the main course. However, don't rush; take your time and enjoy this.

When your partner is ready to offer you the main course, it is time for you to give your love the most pleasure possible while continuing to feast upon this smorgasbord your partner is sharing with you. For the main course, move on to the clitoris, deeper action on the vagina, and the anus. These areas are the most sensitive, and the ones you have been waiting patiently to enjoy. If you have taken your time and stimulated as many of the other areas as possible, your partner will now be ready for you to enjoy these as well.

Now, these areas are most sensitive to many women. The clitoris, while it is often key to oral pleasure for your female partner, it can also become too sensitive to even touch. It can be a YES! YES! YES! and then all of a sudden STOP! kind of scenario, so be prepared for that moment when the pleasure may be too much for her to handle. The other areas, such as the Urethral Opening and the anus, can be amazing pleasure locations for oral sex, but are not usually as hyper-sensitive as the clitoris is. Some people have issues with performing oral sex around the Urethral Opening and the anus because they are also the exit points for urine and feces to exit the body. However, these two areas can be highly arousing when focused on orally.

When feasting on the anus and urethral opening, you can be a little more aggressive in your pursuit. Stimulating these areas with your fingers and mouth prepares them to have your tongue easily start to slide all over them.

Moving to the clitoris is like shoving everything off the table in preparation for that which you have been waiting on. Slowly begin your assault on the deliciousness of the clitoris. Take your time to enjoy the taste, smell, and the texture of the outlying areas. Remember, the clitoris is more than just a little nub. It is an organ that is bigger than you might think, so you can add some hand play around the areas associated with the big picture of the clitoris.

THE STRUCTURE OF THE CLITORIS

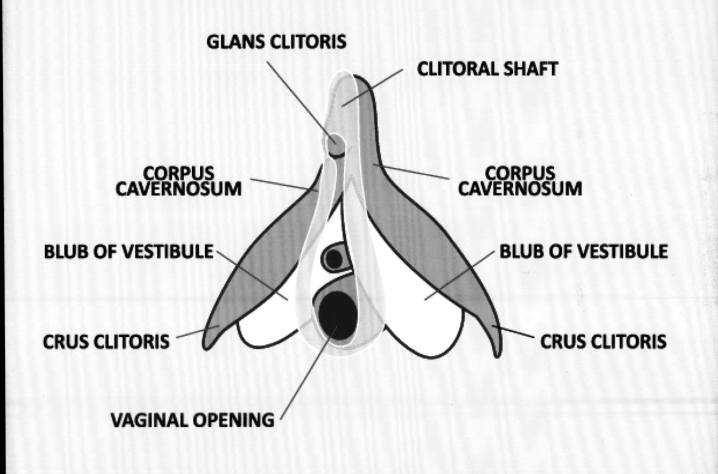

GLANS CLITORIS

CLITORAL SHAFT

CORPUS CAVERNOSUM

CORPUS CAVERNOSUM

BLUB OF VESTIBULE

BLUB OF VESTIBULE

CRUS CLITORIS

CRUS CLITORIS

VAGINAL OPENING

As you tease and play around this palate of amazing delight, the head of the clitoris, the clitoris glans, will begin to swell and become ripe for enjoyment. At this moment, you can move your position to focus on this delicious moment in the feast. Some trial and error will show how your partner responds to different motions and intensities from your tongue and mouth. One thing to try is swirling your tongue around the clitoris, making circles. Start out slowly and then go faster, or to flick your tongue back and forth on your partner's clit, again starting slow and building up. A more advanced technique is to suck the clitoris out from its cover and then stimulate it more. Suck on the clitoris like you were sucking on a straw, not too hard unless encouraged, then once you have pulled it out of hiding, use the swirl or the flick on it at this point.

Trust me, your partner will tell you when their clitoris has had enough. This doesn't mean the feast has to end; you can continue to move back down the original path that led us here, feasting on the love juices that have come into being from this wonderful pleasure.

There are some additional aspects of the feast you should know about. The first being that the taste, smell, and texture of your love can change depending on the point your partner is at in their monthly cycle. Many ancient traditions consider the juices that flow during this process to be sacred and extremely healthy for the partner to consume. Some traditions will also collect the fluids released during these sessions and use them for a variety of things, from anointing items in a spiritual manner, to sharing the juice in rituals of food and dance.

Like in the feasts of old, you might have to take a napkin and wipe the enjoyment from your face, but that just means that you have enjoyed an amazing feast.

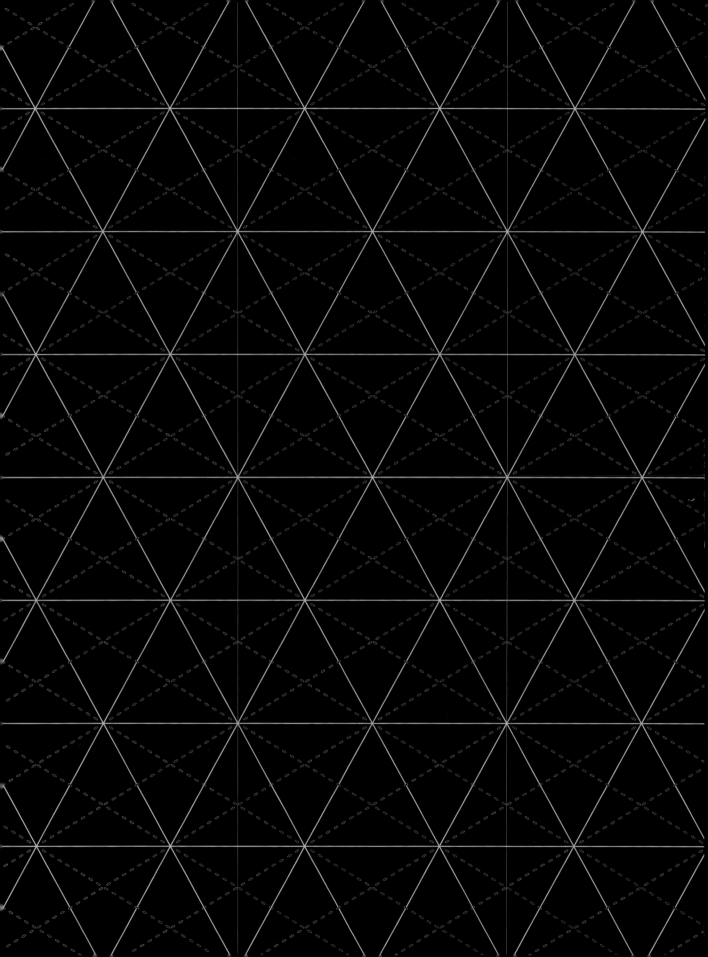

Chapter 5: Oral Sex Positions for Him

ORAL SEX TIPS FOR MEN—SEE ME, FEEL ME

To really please a man with oral sex, not only does it have to physically be good, but visually stimulating as well. When you speak to most men, they will tell you that a big part of the excitement about oral sex is watching their partner perform oral sex on their penis and hearing the sounds they make. When you include visual stimulation alongside the physical pleasures associated with oral sex, you will be able to drive your man wild, and have him begging for more.

Sure, your man wants to have his penis sliding in and out of your mouth, but men also enjoy the foreplay associated with oral sex. Don't just put his penis in your mouth and go to town. Start by slowly caressing his penis with your hands and studying his penis. Let your man watch you admiring his penis and studying it like there will be a test afterwards. Glide your hands all over his penis as you do this, caressing his member to make it as hard as it can become. Take the time to not only study and caress his penis, but to pay careful attention to his scrotum and testicles, as well; they are as much as a part of oral sex as the shaft and head of his penis.

Now that you have your man's attention, and his penis is aroused to an epic erection, it is time to bring in the tongue. Allow your tongue to lick its way up the shaft of his penis, slowly moving up to the head. Once there, pay careful attention to the ridge around the head of the penis, making sure to lick and caress this sensitive area. You should be getting some moans from your partner at this point, which is an excellent sign. Next, use your tongue to caress the head of his penis. You can also flick it a little with your tongue; this will drive your man crazy. You can also put the head of his penis in your mouth from time to time, especially if you notice he is watching.

Only now is it time to start sucking. Here's a little trick that can really drive your man wild, but you have to be careful; some men are way too sensitive to have this done to them. While holding onto the shaft of his penis or caressing the head of his penis, slowly start to lick your way back down to his scrotum. Once you reach his scrotum, open your mouth and gently bring one of his testicles into your mouth. Once his testicle is in your mouth, slowly and gently start to suck on his testicle. Increase the pressure until you can see how much he can take. Believe me, you will know when you reach the "too-much" zone. Be prepared for your man to cry things out at this point, as the pleasure/pain aspects come very close together. Make sure to approach the other testicle with the same process. You might notice that one might be more sensitive than the other, or that your man might be too sensitive for this activity at all; or he may even beg for more!

As you take the pleasure up to a higher level, you have a decision to make. Are you going to take him all the way to orgasm orally or not? There are things to consider here, like the rejuvenation process for a man can be lengthy one, so if you make him climax orally, you might not get his penis inside you for a bit. There is also the concern that some people have about taking a man's ejaculate in their mouth, be it the taste, or just the thought of it. It really is a matter of personal preference and one that you should discuss with your partner. We are going to continue assuming that you are going to make your man climax orally.

Now that you have almost pushed him over the edge sucking on his testicles, move your mouth up to the head of his penis and allow it to enter your mouth. Use the friction from your wet lips (the ones on your face) to lubricate his penis as it slides in and out of your mouth. The size of your man's penis will dictate how much of it you can get into your mouth; if your man is larger, or if your mouth isn't designed to accept all of his penis, you have other options. The most common one is to use your hands to stroke the shaft of his penis, while you focus the oral pleasure on the head of his penis. You can use a straight up-and-down stroke with your hand, or you can kind of twist your wrist to give a corkscrew type of feeling. A very nice touch from time to time while you are stroking his penis, is to take his penis a little deeper in your mouth to mix things up a bit.

As this continues and your man is getting closer to climax, he might start to tell you what is going on with him. Many men like to announce it as they approach climax—one, to warn their partner about the explosion that is about to happen; and two, men just like saying it. If your man is not very vocal, you will notice his penis swelling even more, especially the head of the penis. It may start to throb and release some fluid. You may also sense your man tightening up as he tries to hold onto this pleasure as long as he can.

If you enjoy the flavor of your lover's ejaculate, you can let him fill your mouth with ejaculate without any worries; however, if you are not a big fan of the flavor, you can move his penis more to the back of your throat and allow the ejaculate to quickly move down your throat. And if you just can't stand the flavor, or thought of this fluid being in your mouth, you can always pull it out of your mouth and continue to stroke his penis until he ejaculates from your hand job alone.

BONUS TIPS: These bonus tips will drive most men crazy, and while they are not for everyone, they can create an even more sensual and exciting experience for him.

#1—Make eye contact. This is something that will drive most men totally over the edge if they look down and are met by your beautiful eyes staring back at them while you are licking or sucking on their penis.

#2—Let his orgasm flow all over your face and mouth. This tip is designed for even more visual stimulation, and allows your man to actually see you taking his ejaculate into your mouth. Just as he is about to orgasm, pull his penis out of your mouth and continue to stroke his penis with your hand, allowing him to see his ejaculate coming out of his penis and into your mouth, or onto your mouth area. It will drive your man nuts, as he will get the visual and physical pleasure at the same time.

#3—Use a cock ring on your partner while performing oral sex upon him. This will give a totally different sensation. It will make his erection seem firmer and harder, but it will also slow down the evacuation process, so it might take him little longer to climax. Beware that sometimes this also causes his ejaculate to be a little more pressurized as well, so it might shoot a little farther than normal. So, if you are pulling his penis out of your mouth and finishing him off with a hand job, you might have to duck. The cock ring might also extend his climax a few more moments than normal, but that is a good thing as well.

#4—Use restraints. Lastly, something that may drive your man totally nuts is to do all the actions above, while using restraints on him. You could use an under-the-bed restraint system to allow him to relax on the bed while you pleasure him orally. My suggestion, however, would be to use an over-the-door restraint system to keep him standing up and allow you to have your way with him while he has to observe. He would be unable to stop you from taking him to a pleasure point he most likely has never experienced before.

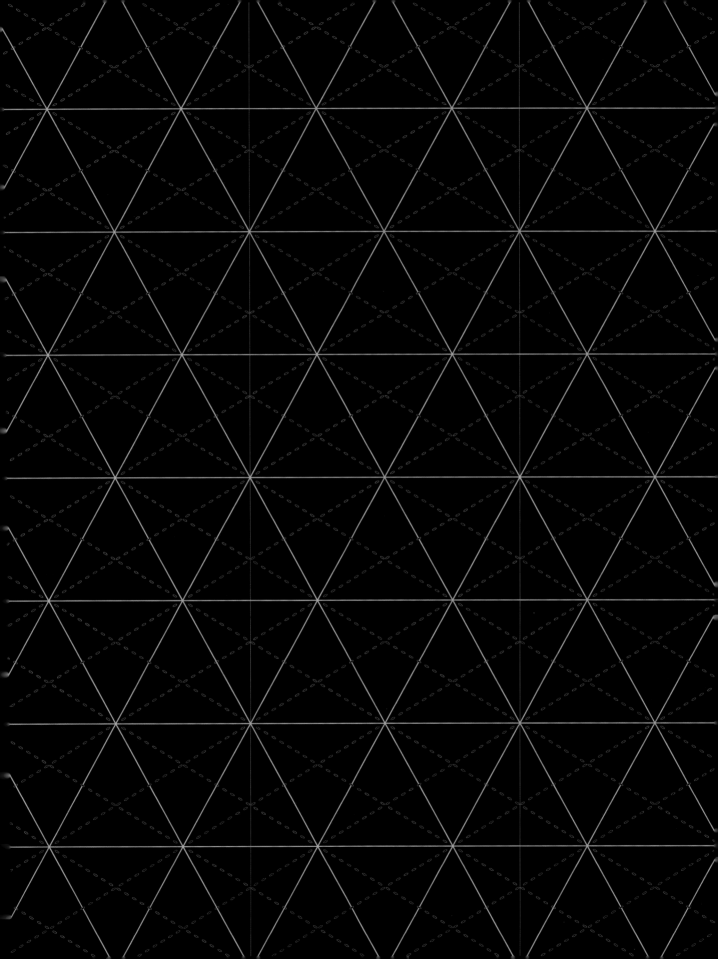

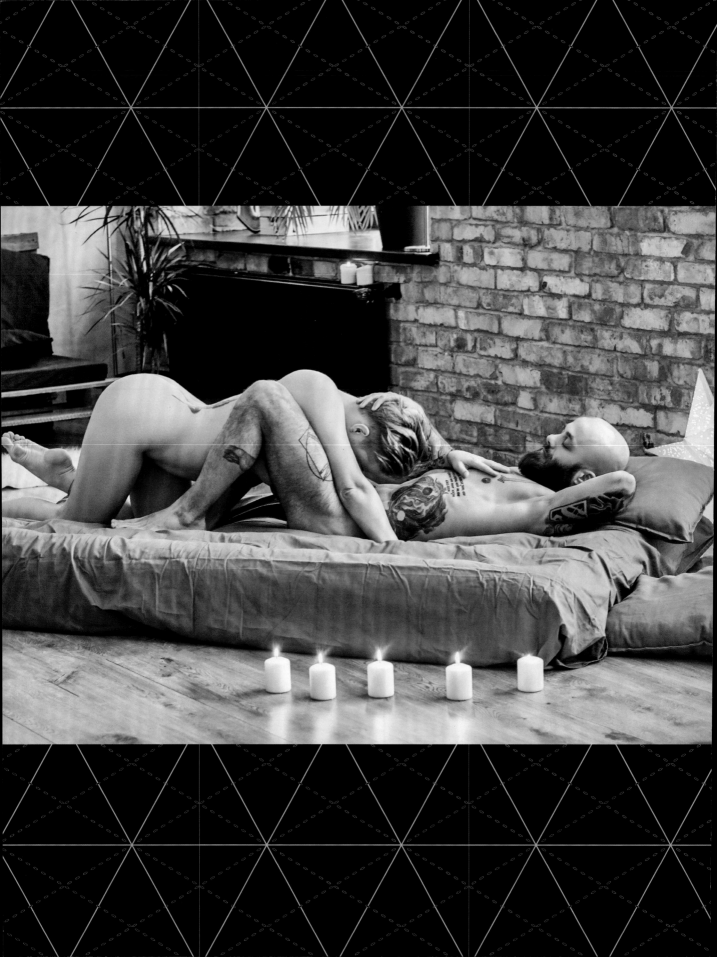

THE ORIGINAL

The "chicken soup" of oral sex positions for him, The Original oral sex position is probably one of his favorite ways to receive a blowjob. It allows him to lie back and relax while he receives pleasure, and it's not terribly difficult for her to do either.

HOW TO DO IT

The male partner lies back, propped up against pillows or even flat on his back, while his partner kneels over him to give oral sex. His legs are spread enough so that she can get in between them, and she can either support her weight on her knees or lie flat on her stomach.

WHERE TO DO IT

The Original oral sex position can be done on the bed, sofa, floor, or perhaps even the car! This is a very versatile oral sex position for both partners. Feel free to do it anywhere you see an opportunity to lie down!

PROPS YOU'LL NEED

He may like some pillows to support his upper torso so he can watch the action.

DIFFICULTY LEVEL ★☆☆☆☆

HER O-METER ★☆☆☆☆

She likes The Original oral sex position because it's easy for her to do, and he enjoys it. This is probably the first oral sex position a woman learns to use!

HIS O-METER ★★★★★

He loves The Original oral sex position simply because it's tried and true. It may be the first kind of blowjob he received, so, of course, there are probably fond memories! He's lying back and relaxing while getting a blowjob, and if he's propped up, he gets to watch. It's simple, yet very, very effective.

MAKE IT HOTTER . . .

Try playing with some submissive roles for her. A sex game where she's "serving" him can be a lot of fun when you incorporate The Original oral sex position in the mix! Or, you can simply revel in the comfort that this oldie, but goodie, gives to both partners.

ALMOST 69

In the Almost-69 oral sex position, he's receiving a blowjob in the same position as 69, but without having to reciprocate. Very hot!

HOW TO DO IT

Both partners lie on their sides, as though they were about to assume the side-by-side 69 sex position, with each partner facing the other's feet. The female partner will proceed to give him oral sex, and while he is in the position to do the same for her, he doesn't. He simply relaxes and enjoys what she's doing to him!

WHERE TO DO IT

The Almost-69 oral sex position can be done in a variety of places, especially narrow ones like the back seat of a car. Since both partners are lying side by side, not as much space is required. Use your imagination here!

PROPS YOU'LL NEED

None.

DIFFICULTY LEVEL ★☆☆☆☆

HER O-METER ★☆☆☆☆

The Almost-69 oral sex position is comfortable for her, but she might just wish he would go down on her at the same time and turn it into a regular 69!

HIS O-METER ★★★★☆

While he does enjoy regular 69, the idea of using the Almost-69 oral sex position is a bonus for him, because he gets to concentrate on his own pleasure, instead of trying to split his concentration between receiving pleasure and giving her oral sex at the same time.

MAKE IT HOTTER . . .

If he wants her to get more out of the Almost-69 position, he can easily use his fingers to stimulate her clitoris, her G-spot, or even her anus if she likes anal play.

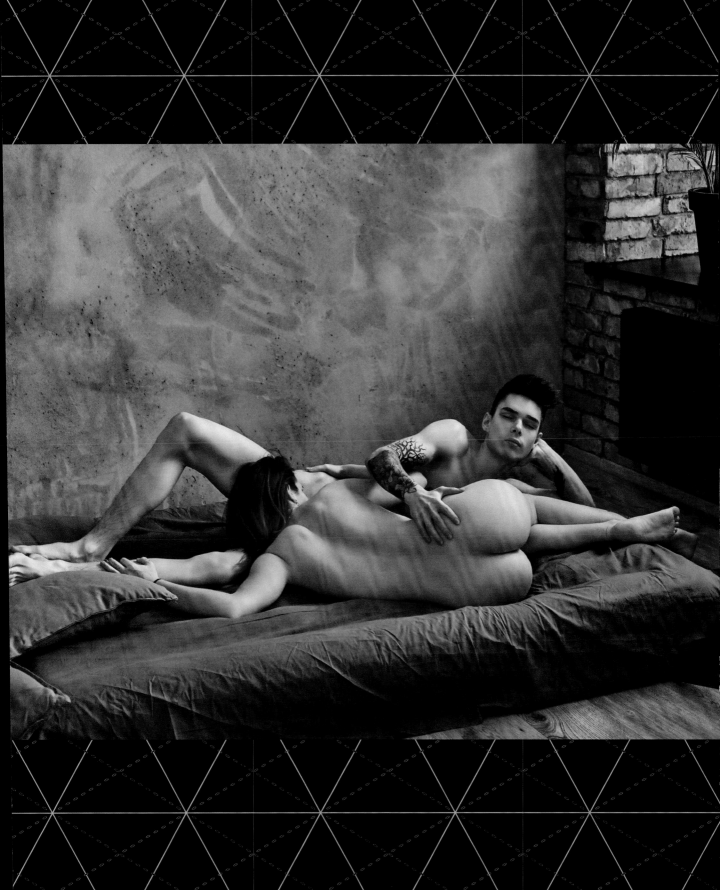

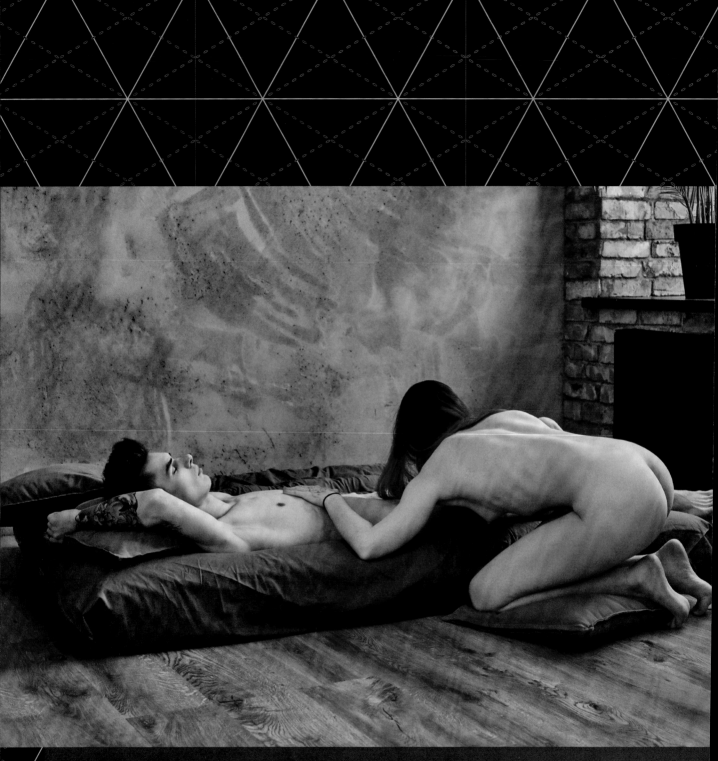

MAKE IT HOTTER...

Ladies, if you reach down and fondle yourself while you're giving your man oral sex in this position, he'll love it. He may not be able to see exactly what you're doing, but he'll really get off on the fact that you're so turned on by going down on him that you can't help but touch yourself! If he's game, this is a great position for a little prostate stimulation to really give him an explosive orgasm!

BLOWJOB THERAPY

Perhaps one of the best oral sex positions for him, Blowjob Therapy allows a man to lie back, relax, and enjoy a blowjob in the utmost comfort. He can lay all the way back and close his eyes, or check her out while she goes down on him. This is truly an oral sex position he will love!

HOW TO DO IT

The Blowjob-Therapy oral sex position is an exceptionally comfortable and enjoyable one for a man. He's laid back on the sofa or the edge of the bed, relaxed and comfortable. His female partner is kneeling at his groin, leaning over the sofa or bed to perform oral sex on him. It's a fairly easy oral sex position to use, and it is much more conducive to the male orgasm than a standing oral sex position, since it can sometimes be difficult for men to ejaculate when they're concentrating on standing and not falling backwards if their knees get weak.

WHERE TO DO IT

This is a perfect position for the sofa, a lounge chair by the pool, or even the edge of a low bed.

PROPS YOU'LL NEED

Pillows under her knees will make it far more enjoyable for her.

DIFFICULTY LEVEL ★☆☆☆☆

HER O-METER ★☆☆☆☆

This oral-sex position is fairly comfortable for the female partner and does reduce neck cramps somewhat, which can be a huge problem when it comes to giving great head. She can also reach down and stimulate herself in this position, making the experience more enjoyable for her.

HIS O-METER ★★★★☆

He's relaxed, he's comfortable, and he's kicking back while getting a blowjob. What's for a man not to love about the Blowjob-Therapy oral sex position? He can lay back and concentrate on the pleasure with his eyes closed, or he can prop his head up on a pillow if he wants to watch the action.

DEEP THROAT

The Deep-Throat oral sex position is definitely a favorite for guys because it creates some of the deepest oral penetration he's ever had during a blowjob!

HOW TO DO IT

The female partner lies on the bed in such a way that her head is draped over the edge of the bed, facing up towards the ceiling. Her partner then kneels and crouches in a way that allows him to penetrate her mouth, resting his weight, and controlling his movements with his arms on the bed. The Deep-Throat oral sex position allows her throat to be elongated so he can penetrate deeply, and it also helps her suppress her gag reflex.

WHERE TO DO IT

The bed is the best place for the Deep-Throat oral sex position!

PROPS YOU'LL NEED

None.

DIFFICULTY LEVEL ★☆☆☆☆

HER O-METER ★☆☆☆☆

If she likes being submissive, the Deep-Throat oral sex position is going to be one of her favorite ways to give her lover a blowjob. If she prefers to be more in control during oral sex, she's not going to like that he is in complete control of how fast and deep he thrusts into her throat.

HIS O-METER ★★★★★

He absolutely loves the Deep-Throat oral sex position. It affords him the deepest oral penetration possible, and allows his penis to be stimulated orally from shaft to tip. He also loves being in control, but he's got to watch how deep and fast he thrusts.

WARNING: A safe gesture is probably a good idea here, so she can easily and quickly let him know if he's hurting her or making her uncomfortable in any way.

MAKE IT HOTTER . . .

She can reach down and stimulate her clitoris with either her hands or a sex toy. He'll love the idea that she's so turned on by the Deep-Throat oral sex position that she can't help herself, and he'll also love being able to look at both himself penetrating her mouth and her stimulating herself to orgasm.

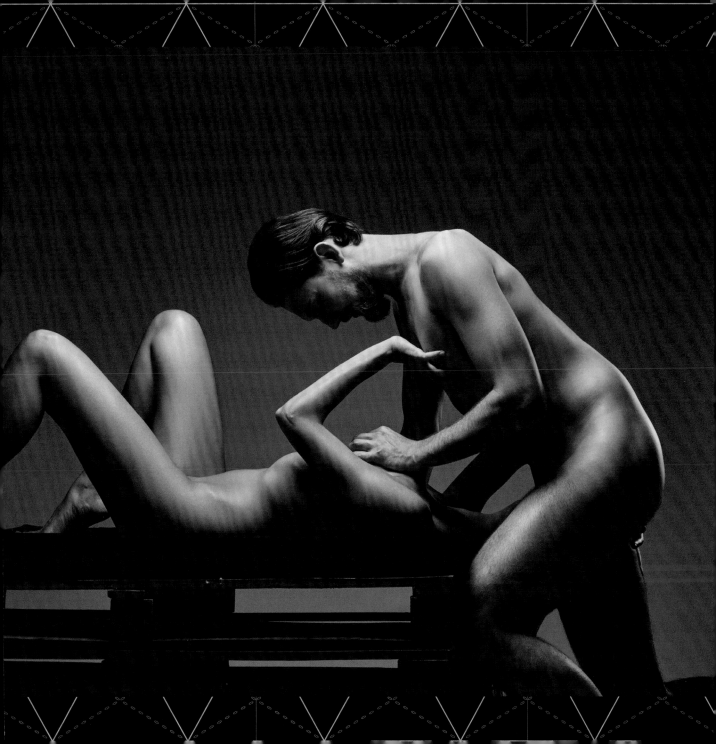

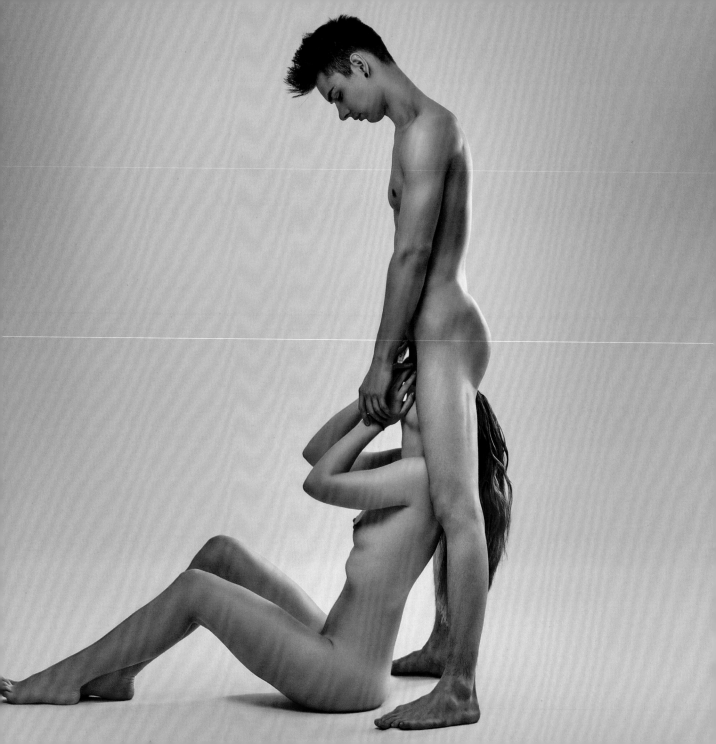

DOWNWARD STROKE

The Downward Stroke is a fun and exciting oral sex position combining a hand job and a blowjob in a way that is comfortable for both him and her. This is a must try!

HOW TO DO IT

The male partner stands with his feet a little wider than shoulder width apart, enough for her to get in between his legs to perform fellatio. The female partner sits on the ground in front of him, facing away from him, and then leans back enough so that her head and mouth are in a good position for oral penetration. She will use her hand to guide his penis into her mouth, and also to stroke the base of his shaft while she sucks on the head. He can also move up and down by bending his knees.

WHERE TO DO IT

The Downward-Stroke oral sex position is an easy one to use on the go, simply because all it requires is for the guy to drop his drawers. So for a quickie blowjob in the bathroom, or in the closet at a friend's house during a party, this sex position is great. Of course, it's also good for home use, and still fun if you're completely naked.

PROPS YOU'LL NEED

None.

DIFFICULTY LEVEL ★☆☆☆☆

HER O-METER ★☆☆☆☆

The Downward-Stroke oral sex position is simple for her to get into, but it's bound to give her quite the crick in the neck.

HIS O-METER ★★★★☆

He loves the combination of oral and manual stimulation in the Down-ward-Stroke oral sex position! This is a great one for guys who have trouble reaching orgasm during oral sex alone, because the heavier stimulation can bring them to climax much more easily and quickly.

MAKE IT HOTTER . . .

She can use her other hand to stimulate her clitoris or to use a sex toy, which will give him an awesome show to enjoy while she's performing oral sex!

FACE STRADDLE FOR HIM

The Face Straddle for Him is a primal, sexy way for her to submit during oral sex for him. He loves how animalistic this sex position is!

HOW TO DO IT

The male partner gets on all fours, and the female partner lies down on her back, with her knees bent and her feet flat with her head underneath her partner's hips. This allows him to bend down slightly and penetrate her mouth and throat with his penis from above. She can grasp his hips and buttocks and pull herself up to him, or pull him down to her.

WHERE TO DO IT

Due to the amount of space required by this position, it is much easier to do this on a bed. However, it can be done on the sofa or floor, but it isn't as comfortable.

PROPS YOU'LL NEED

A pillow under her head will not only make her more comfortable, but it will lift her head and neck some to help her reach him without having to strain so much.

DIFFICULTY LEVEL ★☆☆☆☆

HER O-METER ★☆☆☆☆

The Face Straddle for Him may be one of her favorites if she likes for him to have control of the thrusting during a blowjob, but if she doesn't, she won't like it very much. If he thrusts too fast or too hard, it may be uncomfortable or painful for her, and she may have difficult time breathing.

WARNING: A safe gesture in this case is an exceptionally good idea, so she can quickly and easily let him know if he needs to stop because he's making her uncomfortable, or she can't breathe very well.

HIS O-METER ★★★★★

He enjoys how submissive his partner is in this position and how in control he is over the thrusting. He also likes how "primal" it feels with him on all fours!

MAKE IT HOTTER . . .

If he enjoys having his prostate stimulated, or even if he just enjoys a little anal play, she can easily reach around and use her hands to give him some naughty pleasure.

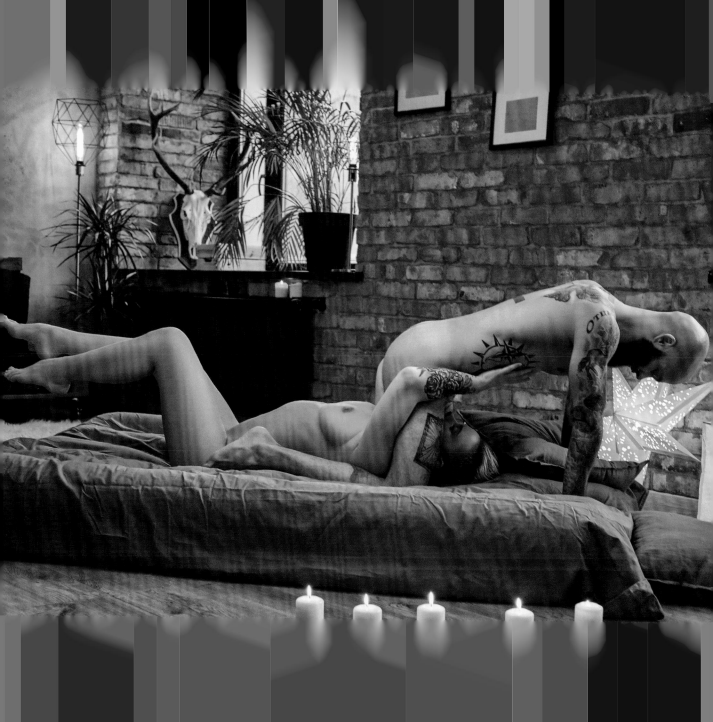

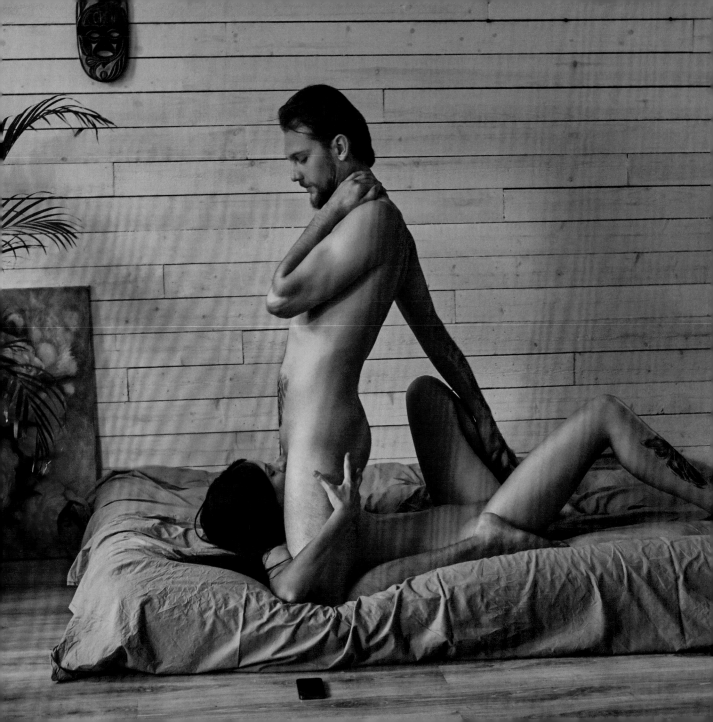

FACE THRUST

If he likes being in control, the Face-Thrust oral sex position is an incredible turn on for him, but some women may find it a little uncomfortable.

HOW TO DO IT

The female partner lies on her back on a surface, with her head propped up by a pillow. The male partner straddles her chest on his knees, bringing his penis close to her face. He can grasp her head and use it to help him thrust in and out of her mouth. The female partner does very little in the Face-Thrust oral sex position.

WHERE TO DO IT

A bed is surely to be the most comfortable place for this sex position; however, it can be done on the sofa, or even on the floor if her head has enough support.

PROPS YOU'LL NEED

You'll need one or two pillows under her head and neck for support, and to raise her head enough for penetration.

DIFFICULTY LEVEL ★☆☆☆☆

HER O-METER ★☆☆☆☆

The Face Thrust oral sex position is probably not going to be her very favorite, simply because it can be quite uncomfortable for her. It's easy to get a neck cramp in this position, and since her partner is in total control, she has no say over how fast she gives him head or how deep the thrusting goes. This can easily lead to gagging and difficulty breathing.

WARNING: It's a good idea to develop a safe gesture she can use to let him know if he's getting too freaky, or if she's uncomfortable in any way. Both partners need to agree that if the safe gesture is used, the action stops immediately.

HIS O-METER ★★★★★

Most guys love the idea of being in total control of a blowjob, even if they don't get to actually do it very often. In the Face-Thrust oral sex position, he can hold her head while he thrusts in and out of her mouth, which is a huge fantasy for a lot of men. He totally digs this sex position!

MAKE IT HOTTER . . .

Since her hands are free, she can use them to caress his lower back and buttocks. If he likes anal play, she can gently play with this area using her fingers, or even massage his prostate gland. Just use lots of lube first!

HANDSTAND

The Handstand oral sex position is an oral sex position for him that is challenging, yet very exciting if he can pull it off! This is for adventurous couples only.

HOW TO DO IT

The male partner does a handstand on the floor, with his legs straight up in the air. The female partner kneels in front of him, facing his groin, so she can perform oral sex on him.

WHERE TO DO IT

The Handstand oral sex position is one you should try in the safety of your home. There's a definite possibility of falling! He'll probably want to do it on the floor, as he won't be able to support himself on the bed or other soft surface.

PROPS YOU'LL NEED

He may want to lean with his back against the wall for more support as he's doing the handstand. She may be more comfortable with a pillow under her knees.

DIFFICULTY LEVEL ★★★★★

HER O-METER ★☆☆☆☆

She'll like the fact that it's him getting into the wacky position instead of her, because it's almost always the other way around!

HIS O-METER ★☆☆☆☆

If he can pull off the Handstand oral sex position, it's pretty fun for him. The blood rush to his head can make it more pleasurable, but on the other hand, he may find it difficult to maintain a strong erection with the blood going in the opposite direction. Also, the angle of his penis is a bit unnatural, so she definitely needs to be gentle here and not go too fast.

MAKE IT HOTTER . . .

Don't worry about trying to spice up the Handstand oral sex position. This one is plenty hot on its own, if you can actually do it!

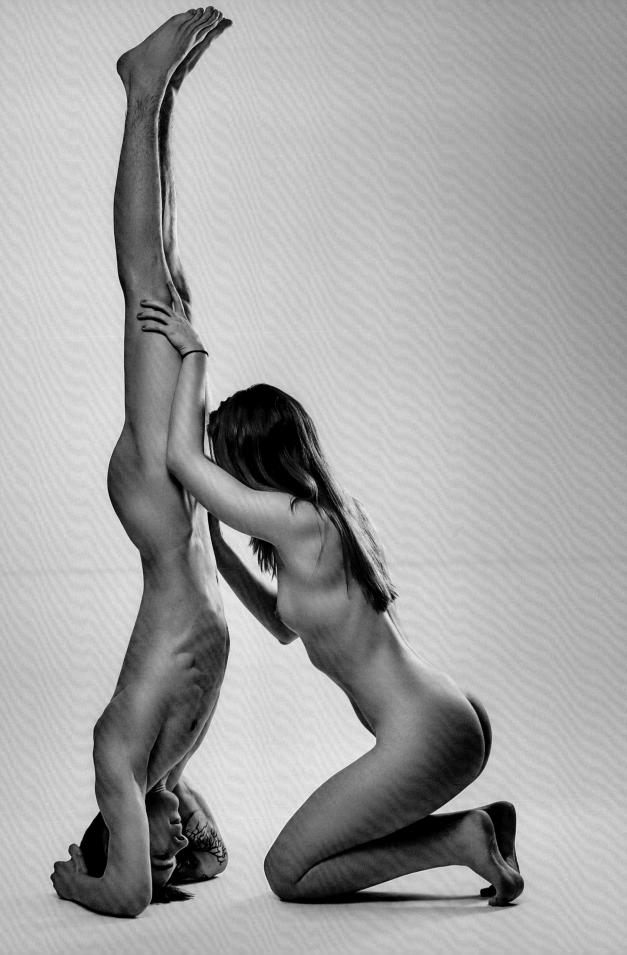

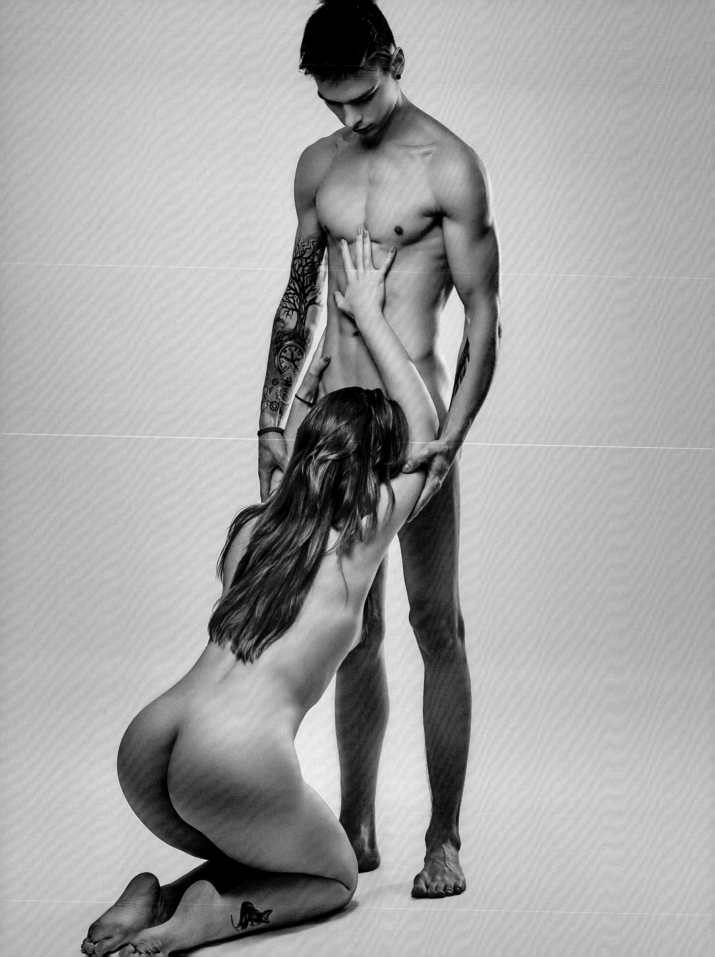

KNEELING BLOWJOB

The Kneeling Blowjob is perhaps one of the most popular oral sex positions for him, and it's definitely one of his favorites. He loves being able to look down and see her going to work on him. If she's really good at it, she might make him weak in the knees! Keep a chair nearby!

HOW TO DO IT

The Kneeling Blowjob is one of the most common oral sex positions for him. It's an extremely powerful position, and he will feel very dominant when he receives a blowjob this way. In this position, the male partner is standing, and the female partner is kneeling in front of him to perform oral sex. This is a very simple, yet effective, oral sex position for him, although some men won't be able to orgasm well in this position because they are standing and cannot relax. Ladies, if you're good enough to make him weak in the knees, you might want to switch to a sitting oral sex position for the finish!

WHERE TO DO IT

Anywhere he can stand is a good place for Kneeling Blowjob!

PROPS YOU'LL NEED

She will greatly appreciate a pillow or folded blanket to slip under her knees.

DIFFICULTY LEVEL ★☆☆☆☆

HER O-METER ★☆☆☆☆

This position can help reduce neck cramps when the female partner is giving oral sex, but may be uncomfortable due to extended periods of time spent on her knees.

HIS O-METER ★★★★★

He loves getting head this way because it makes him feel very manly, as though the female partner is submitting to him—and in a way, she is. He'll enjoy looking down and watching his lover give him oral sex, and making eye contact with her when she looks up after doing her job.

MAKE IT HOTTER . . .

This is an excellent "quickie blowjob" oral sex position. He can drop his drawers almost anywhere, at any time, and if you have enough privacy (and sometimes if you don't) she can suck him off quickly. It's a standard oral sex position that you can make very, very naughty if you get creative!

PEEK-A-BOO

An interesting twist on oral sex for him, the Peek-a-Boo oral sex position is something fun to try when you want something different, but not too exotic.

HOW TO DO IT

The male partner lies on his side on the bed, and his partner lies perpendicular to him, with the majority of her body behind him. He spreads his legs slightly, and she brings her head up to his groin from behind, resting the weight of her head on his inner thigh.

WHERE TO DO IT

Because of the space required for the Peek-a-Boo oral sex position, the bed or floor is your best bet. However, the bed is going to be infinitely more comfortable for both partners!

PROPS YOU'LL NEED

A few pillows for him will help prop his head up and make him more comfortable.

DIFFICULTY LEVEL ★☆☆☆☆

HER O-METER ★☆☆☆☆

The Peek-a-Boo is a comfortable position for her to be in, and it helps prevent neck cramps. This is a big plus for her, because it means she can continue giving oral sex for a significant period of time. She also has partial control here, and if he doesn't use his hand on her head, she'll have full control of the depth and speed of penetration.

HIS O-METER ★★★★☆

He enjoys the Peek-a-Boo oral sex position because it allows him to grasp her head and thrust if he wants, or just lie back and enjoy the sensations! He digs looking down and seeing just her head "peeking" out from in between his legs.

MAKE IT HOTTER . . .

Since her hands are free in the Peek-a-Boo oral sex position, she can easily either give him some anal stimulation if he's into it, or reach down and stimulate herself with her fingers or a sex toy so she gets some pleasure out of it, too!

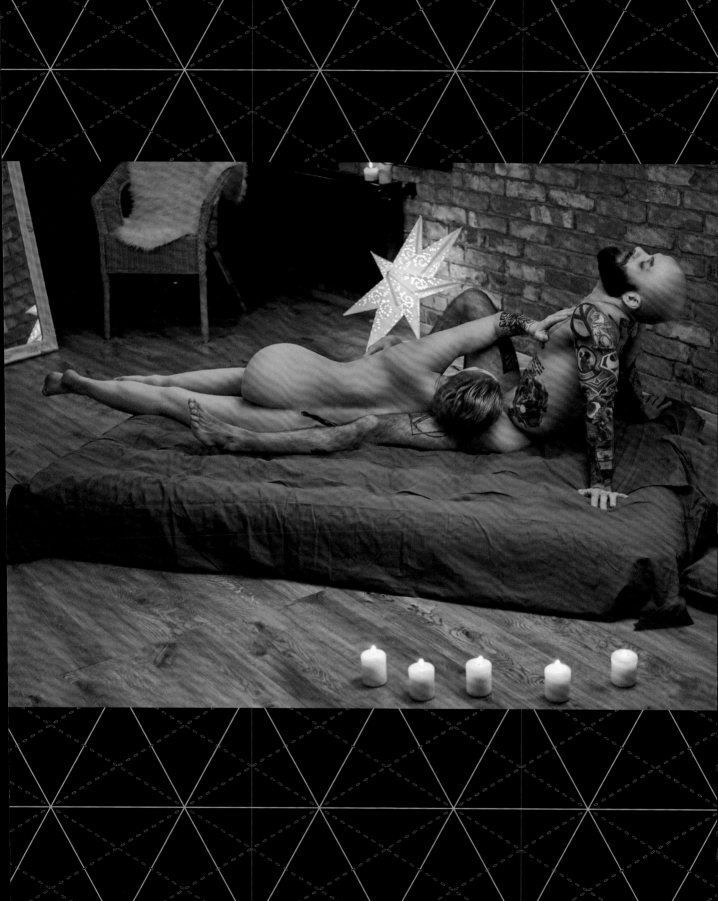

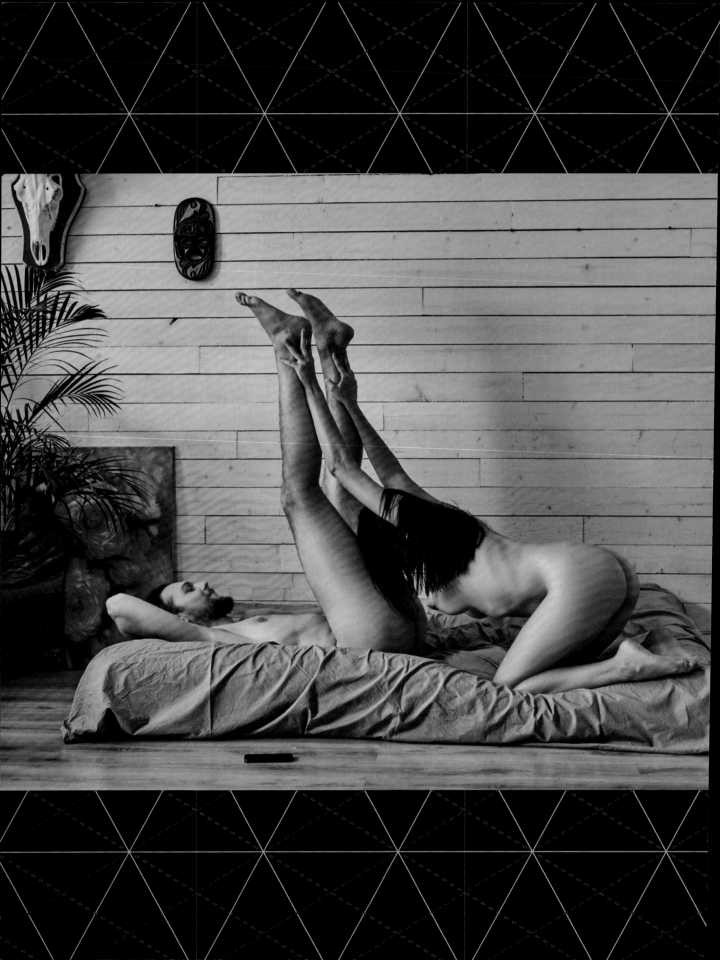

Under the Hood (For Him)

The Under the Hood is one that gives his partner full access to his nether region, and makes him feel exceptionally vulnerable.

HOW TO DO IT

The male partner lies on his back, and brings his legs and knees as close to his chest as possible. Typically, his legs are stretched out, but if this is difficult for him to do, a slight bend in the knees is okay. He can hold the backs of his thighs to help support his legs. The female partner then kneels to give her partner oral sex.

WHERE TO DO IT

A wide space like the bed or floor is best for this position, but the bed is of course going to be much more comfortable.

PROPS YOU'LL NEED

He will want a pillow under his head, and she'll want one under her knees, if she's on the floor. A rolled-up blanket or towel will also work.

DIFFICULTY LEVEL ★☆☆☆☆

HER O-METER ★☆☆☆☆

She likes this position because it turns the tables by giving him the opportunity to feel vulnerable, and her the opportunity to be in complete control.

HIS O-METER ★★★☆☆

If he's not comfortable with his anal area being exposed, he's not going to like this sex position very much. However, for guys who are totally comfortable with themselves, this one is a must try! It's totally hot!

MAKE IT HOTTER . . .

If he enjoys prostate massage, or even a little anilingus during oral sex, the Under the Hood is the perfect position to do it.

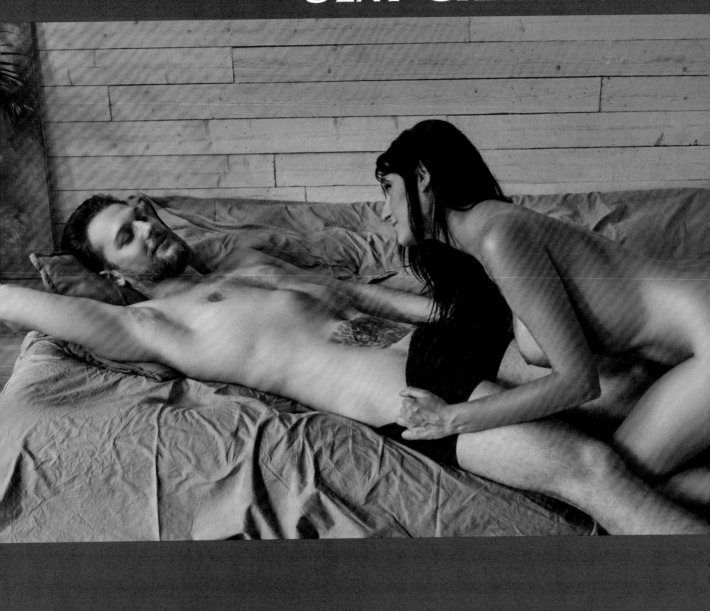

To Boldly Try Something New in Oral Sex For Men

Oral sex for men seems pretty straightforward: insert penis in mouth, and move mouth up and down the penis. However, we challenge you ladies to boldly go in a new direction to add variety and maximize his pleasure. There are many things you can do to add an exciting twist to the standard version of oral sex, and we want to share those bold ideas with you. We are going to give you some fun new strategies to help create a whole new world of oral sex delight for your partner.

LUBRICATE, LUBRICATE, AND LUBRICATE. Saliva is often the lubrication used during oral sex on a man. While this is perfectly fine, there are other options. There are many flavored lubes out there that can help create a different experience for the giver during oral sex on him. Many sexual lubricants might not taste very good, so try out a few different ones to see which ones work best for you. Flavored lubes and coconut oil are great options. There are also heating and cooling lubes that will give your man an entirely different sensation while you please him orally. There are even lubes that glow in the dark to brighten up the experience to a new level.

PUT A RING ON IT. One simple, yet amazing, way to change up the experience of oral sex is to use cock rings to change the sensation. For most guys, a cock ring will delay and extend the orgasm they will have, allowing for those few extra seconds of ejaculatory bliss. You can use a cock ring at the base of the penis, in the middle of the shaft, or right below the head of the penis. Each placement will change the sensations he receives. You can even use multiple cock rings to make things really hot.

HOLD IT NOW. For many men, when they start to climax, the testicles draw up into or towards the body. There are devices available designed to keep the testicles down and allow for more powerful ejaculations. Many of these products are very detailed and complicated. However, once you try this as either the giver or receiver, you will notice a huge difference not only in volume, but in pure pleasure as well.

RAISING YOUR VIBRATION. We associate vibrators with women most often; however, using a vibrator on your man while you are performing oral sex on him can create double the pleasure for him. You can use the vibrator on his testicles and scrotum as you pleasure him orally, or you even to stimulate his anus. Our friends at Hot Octopuss even make a product that will allow you to vibrate the shaft of the penis, while still orally pleasuring the head, and that, my friends, is out-of-this-world pleasure.

HOLDING HIM BACK. Another magical treat you can bring to the pleasuring of your man is to use some restraints on him. Restraining his arms and legs while you bring him to climax orally is most likely to give him an orgasm like never before. When the pleasure of the orgasm gets too amazing, men will often reach down to stop the intense pleasure from continuing, but with a restraint system, the man will be unable to stop the action, thusly taking his pleasure to another level entirely. Any time you use restraints on your partner, make sure to create a safe word or gesture that he can use if the pleasure gets to be too much.

DON'T FORGET THE MUSIC AND LIGHTS. Not all items that intensify the oral sex experience have to be directly related to the penis of a man. Playing music in the background can change the mood of the experience, as can changing the color of the lights. Any stimuli you introduce to the senses during the oral sex experience will alter the feeling and could create more pleasure. This experience might just change the song that you call, "Your Song."

POSITIONS, POSITIONS, POSITIONS. Don't forget the main subject of this book, and consider all the oral sex positions for him listed and shown in the book. You don't always have to be down between your partner's legs to perform oral sex. Make it a point to try all the different oral sex positions listed in this book, and see which ones you and your partner like the best. Make use of any sexual furniture you have, and the liberator ramp and wedge can be a huge help here as well, allowing your partner just to be in a different angle to watch and enjoy.

Performing oral sex on your male partner is like having a conversation. You want this conversation to be exciting and attention-grabbing, as well as leaving your partner craving more! There are some metaphysical traditions that suggest that men can actually breathe through the penis, so performing oral sex might be metaphorically life-giving to your male partner, allowing them a better connection not only with you, but with their soul and their inner self.

CHAPTER 6: SITTING SEX POSITIONS

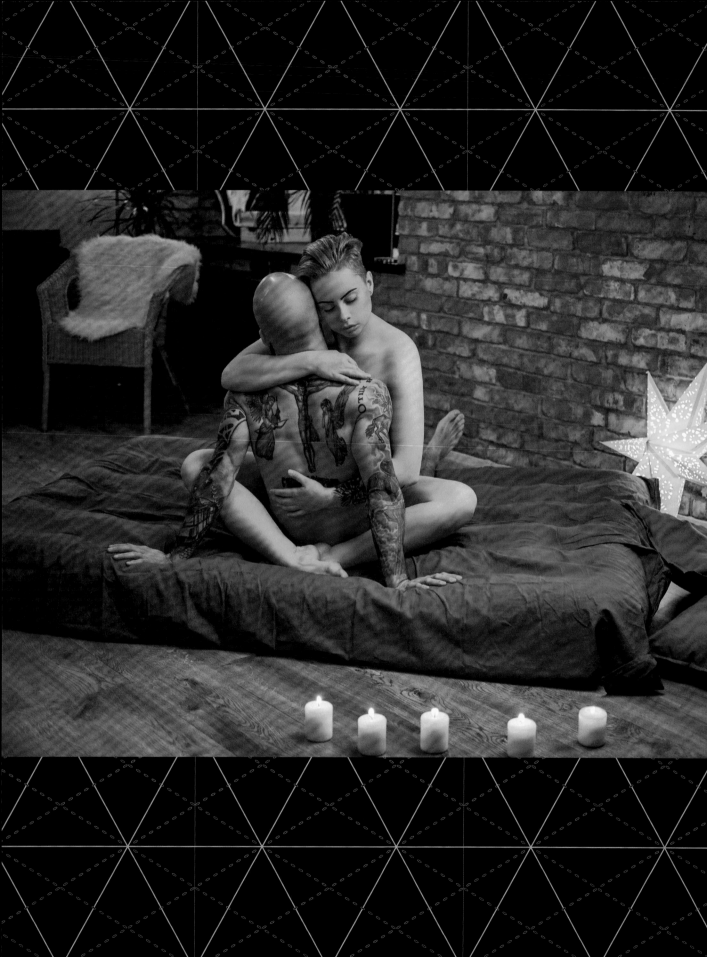

LOTUS

If you want to experience the utmost intimacy with your partner during sex, the Lotus sex position is definitely the way to go. When you're relaxed and sitting with each other, you can slowly rock back and forth, and gradually work your way up to an intense orgasm!

HOW TO DO IT

The Lotus is probably the most intimate sex position out there. If you want to fully connect with your partner emotionally and physically during sex, the Lotus is the way to do it. Both partners sit cross-legged facing each other, but the female partner will actually sit on her lover's lap with her legs wrapped around his hips, so their pelvises touch. Once in position, it is more difficult to "thrust." Sex in the Lotus position involves more "rocking" than it does thrusting. This is what makes the Lotus one of the more unique sex positions that isn't as difficult to achieve!

WHERE TO DO IT

Try the Lotus on the floor, bed, large rocking recliner, or anywhere you have enough space.

PROPS YOU'LL NEED

If you're doing this one on the floor, you'll want a soft blanket or large pillow to prevent carpet burn!

DIFFICULTY LEVEL ★★★☆☆

HER O-METER ★★★★★

Women love the Lotus sex position! Not only does she get an extra dose of the physical and emotional intimacy she craves, the rocking and pelvic grinding does an excellent job of stimulating both her clitoris and her G-spot. This is definitely a position that she can orgasm in!

HIS O-METER ★★★★☆

If he's the sensitive type, he's going to like the emotional connection he gets out of the Lotus, too. Men generally dig anything their partners are into, simply because they're psyched to have a partner who is actually enjoying herself. The rocking motion, however, will put pressure on his penis in a different way, making it feel unique and extra pleasurable for him.

MAKE IT HOTTER . . .

He should give her oral sex before getting into this incredibly intimate sex position. She will literally explode on top of him!

ASSISTED LOTUS

If you have trouble with the Lotus position but still crave face-to-face intimacy, try the Assisted-Lotus sex position. It's easier, and just as sensual.

HOW TO DO IT

The male partner will sit in a chair with his feet on the floor. The female partner will straddle his lap while facing him, and drape each of her legs over the side of the chair. She can wrap her arms around his torso for more stability during thrusting.

WHERE TO DO IT

This is a great one to do in a dining room if you're alone, or any time you spot a chair without arms. It's perfect for a quickie if you don't want to get caught, or a more sensual sex session.

PROPS YOU'LL NEED

You can use a dining room chair or any other chair that has no arms.

DIFFICULTY LEVEL ★☆☆☆☆

HER O-METER ★★★★

There's nothing about the Assisted-Lotus sex position that she doesn't like. She loves the face-to-face intimacy, she loves the comfort of doing it on a chair instead of on the bed, and she loves the clitoral friction. This is a very easy sex position for her to reach orgasm in, because it provides the emotional and physical stimulation she needs to climax.

HIS O-METER ★★★★☆

He too enjoys the intimacy here, and although he can't thrust in and out as well as he can in other sex positions, the rocking and grinding motions that the Assisted-Lotus sex position affords are quite pleasurable. It's a great sex position for a man who doesn't want to orgasm too fast during sex, and wants her to reach orgasm first.

MAKE IT HOTTER...

Make out! Kiss and caress your lover with your mouth the entire time. Engaging this often-forgotten sexual organ can really fire the Assisted-Lotus sex position up!

To take this in another direction, blindfold him and ties his hands behind the chair with a neck tie. This will awaken all of his other senses!

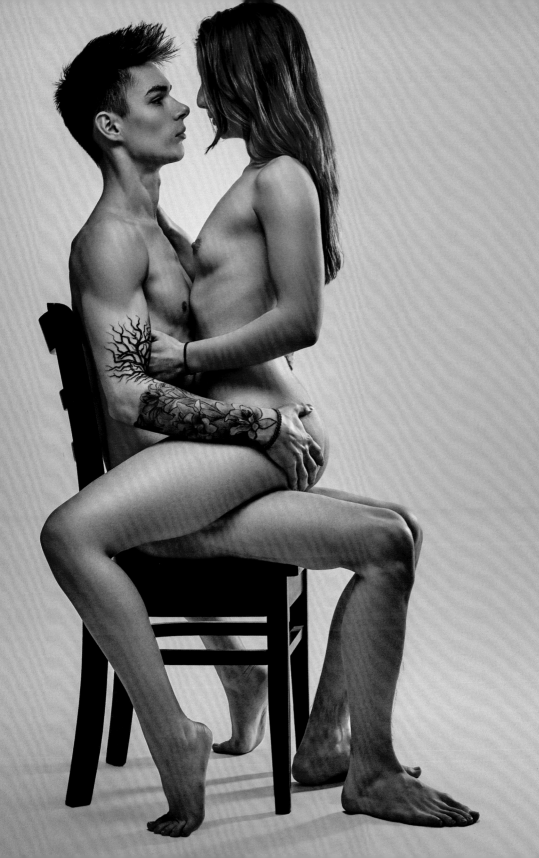

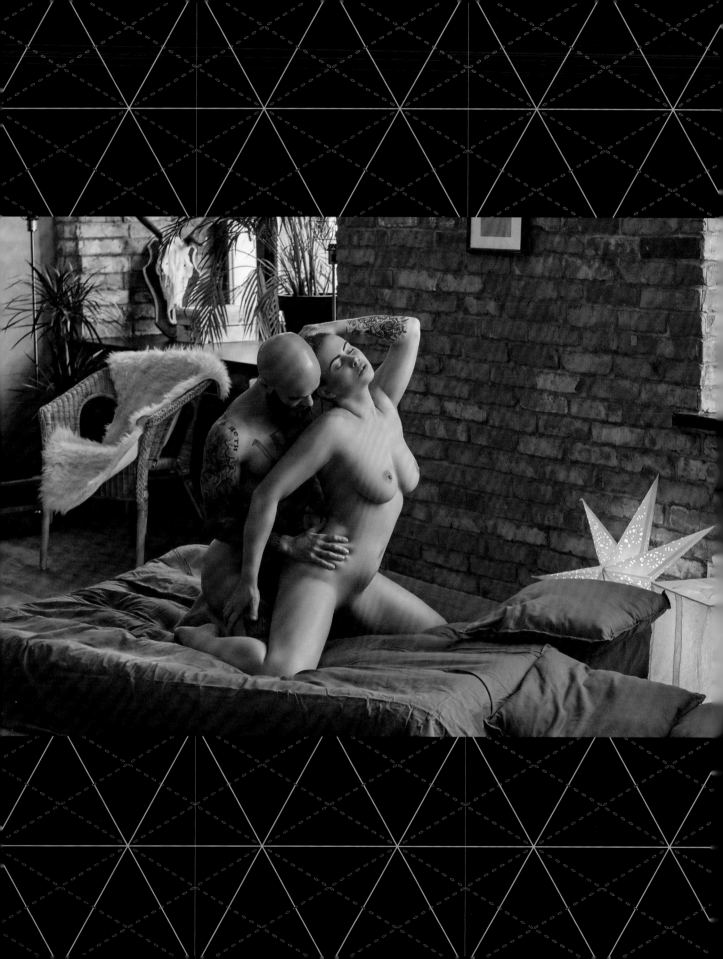

KNEELING EMBRACE

The Kneeling-Embrace sex position is a sweet and sensual combination of sitting, rear entry, and woman on top that is orgasmic for both partners.

HOW TO DO IT

In the Kneeling-Embrace sex position, the male partner sits on a flat surface on his knees, with his knees together or spread only slightly apart. The female partner sits in a similar manner on top of her partner's lap, facing away from him. Her knees are spread slightly to give her lover better access to her vagina.

WHERE TO DO IT

While you can do the Kneeling-Embrace sex position on the floor, it's going to be hard on your knees if you choose to do so. You'll want the comfort and space of a bed or folded-down futon. This could, however, be a fun sex position to try outdoors on a soft bed of grass!

PROPS YOU'LL NEED

None.

DIFFICULTY LEVEL ★☆☆☆☆

HER O-METER ★☆☆☆☆

If her lover has a smaller penis, the penetration isn't going to be as deep in this sex position as others. However, she may enjoy the unique intimacy here, and the fact that he can reach around and fondle her breasts or clitoris.

HIS O-METER ★★★☆☆

Because his legs are pressed together, his entire penile shaft isn't going to get stimulated here, so the Kneeling-Embrace sex position may not be his favorite. However, he'll enjoy caressing and kissing his partner's back as she grinds and thrusts against him.

MAKE IT HOTTER . . .

Either partner can reach forward and stimulate her clitoris for more orgasm potential for her, or if you're fairly adventurous, you might also want to try anal sex in the Kneeling-Embrace sex position. This may work better for women who are new to anal sex, since penetration isn't quite as deep as with other anal sex positions.

LAP DANCE

The Lap Dance is a fun rear-entry sex position, but can lack intimacy due to the way each partner is facing. Thrusting can also be a little difficult, but he can have a lot of fun playing with her breasts while she rides him. It can also be a great follow-up sex position to a real lap dance!

HOW TO DO IT

This is another rear-entry sex position, but it happens to be a little more difficult than some of the others. In this sex position, the male partner is seated on a surface such as the edge of the bed, sofa, or a chair with his feet flat on the floor. The female partner lowers herself onto him, facing away from him with her back against his chest. That sounds easy enough, but the difficult part of this sex position is getting the female partner's feet in position—her feet are tucked behind her, facing away from her on either side of her partner's body. This can be an awkward position if a woman is not very flexible.

WHERE TO DO IT

A sofa, bed, or chair is best for Lap Dance, but anywhere that allows the male partner to sit on the edge with his feet on the floor will work in a pinch.

PROPS YOU'LL NEED

Sofa, bed, or chair.

DIFFICULTY LEVEL ★★★★☆

HER O-METER ★☆☆☆☆

This sex position is more difficult for her to get into and stay in than her partner. It can be a little awkward, especially since the thrusting is mainly her responsibility. This is where it can get tough, because she's going to have to raise up on her shins, and most women aren't used to maneuvering that way during sex. It can take some time getting used to how to move to create the best penetration.

HIS O-METER ★★★☆☆

Since he's in a natural sitting position, with her facing away from him and sitting on his lap, this sex position isn't really that uncomfortable for him. He doesn't have a view, though, unless he and his lover are getting it on in front of a mirror.

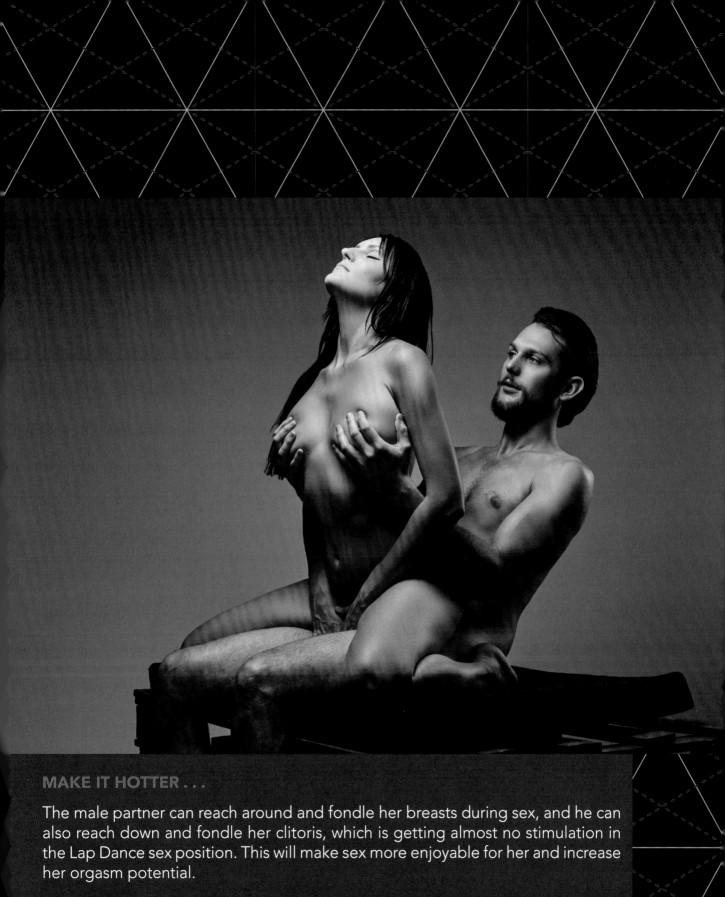

MAKE IT HOTTER . . .

The male partner can reach around and fondle her breasts during sex, and he can also reach down and fondle her clitoris, which is getting almost no stimulation in the Lap Dance sex position. This will make sex more enjoyable for her and increase her orgasm potential.

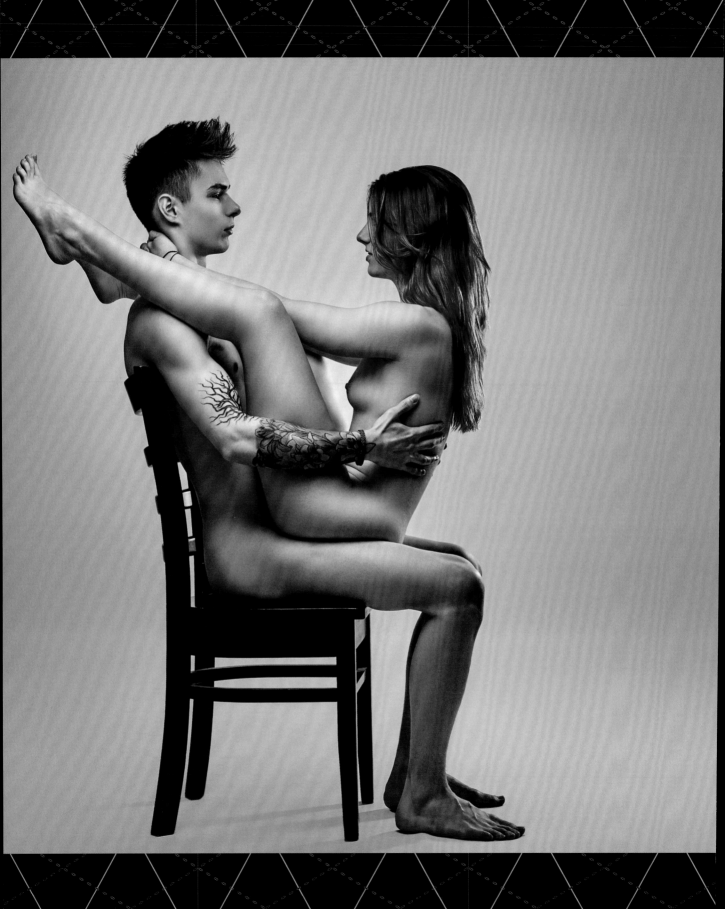

LAPTOP

The Laptop sex position is an interesting variation on the Assisted Lotus (see page 144), and although it looks difficult, it's really not. It's definitely a must try!

HOW TO DO IT

The male partner sits in a chair with his feet flat on the floor, while his lover sits on his lap, facing him. Instead of wrapping her legs on either side of the chair, she will rest the backs of her knees on her partner's shoulders, and her calves and feet on the back of the chair. She can grasp his neck to help maintain her balance, but he should be holding her lower back to help keep her steady.

WHERE TO DO IT

This is an awesome sex position for a quickie at the office, or anywhere else you see a chair and an opportunity!

PROPS YOU'LL NEED

Almost any chair will work, but for the Laptop sex position, you may want to use a more comfortable chair, like a recliner or a nice office chair.

DIFFICULTY LEVEL ★★★☆☆

HER O-METER ★★★☆☆

She enjoys the deep penetration that the Laptop sex position affords, because it's perfect for G-spot stimulation. Some women may need more clitoral stimulation to orgasm than this position can give, but it's still a great one to try.

HIS O-METER ★★★☆☆

He loves the feeling of his partner's legs around his neck, and enjoys the deep penetration sensations. The Laptop sex position is perfect for "breast guys," since he is eye level with her chest!

MAKE IT HOTTER . . .

The male partner can really focus on her breasts here, caressing them with his lips and tongue. This will help her to reach orgasm even faster too!

PRETZEL

The Pretzel sex position is a seated sex position that creates intimacy between both partners with its face-to-face rocking and grinding.

HOW TO DO IT

To get into the Pretzel sex position, the male partner must sit on a flat surface and lie back while resting his weight on his hands behind him. His lover will then straddle him, lowering herself onto his penis. She grasps the back of her thighs, and holds her legs up with her knees slightly parted, so her partner can come in between them. The male partner then sits up so he is face-to-face with her. As he sits up, he will hook his legs over her arms and around her body, completing the "pretzel" configuration.

WHERE TO DO IT

The bed is your best bet for the Pretzel sex position. This is a difficult position to get into and maneuver in, so you'll want the comfort and familiarity of your bed.

PROPS YOU'LL NEED

None.

DIFFICULTY LEVEL ★★★★★

HER O-METER ★☆☆☆☆

She'll like the face-to-face intimacy of the Pretzel sex position, but that's about it. This isn't going to be on her "favorites" list, and it's probably not one she'll suggest trying. She might be on board if her lover is really into exotic sex, but the penetration isn't very deep here, and her clitoris isn't adequately stimulated for her to be able to build a good orgasm.

HIS O-METER ★☆☆☆☆

He likes the novelty of this sex position, but his penis is bent at a slightly awkward angle and thrusting is fairly difficult here. It's mostly a rock and grind sort of motion. He'll want to try this move for sure, because it's so exotic, but it's not going to be one he does regularly.

MAKE IT HOTTER . . .

Focus more on actually getting into the Pretzel sex position than on making it hotter. You're doing well if you can get in it and actually have sex for more than a few minutes!

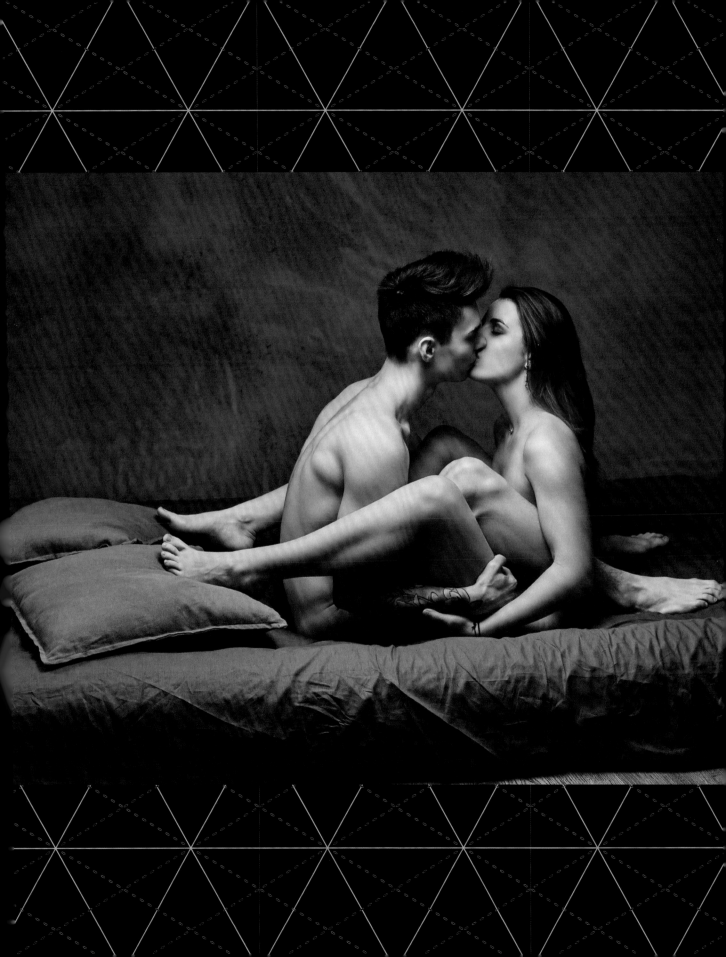

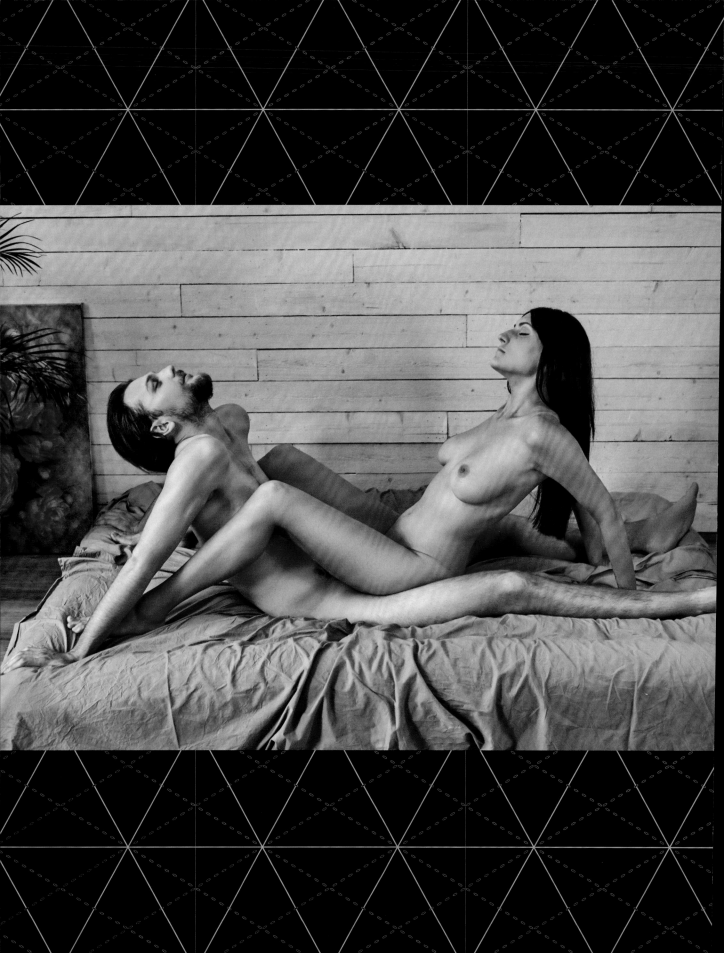

SEESAW

Express your intimacy and achieve intense orgasms with the Seesaw sex position. This is an easy one to do that both partners really enjoy!

HOW TO DO IT

The male partner sits on the floor or the bed, with his legs stretched out and supporting his weight on his arms behind him. She straddles him, facing him, with her feet flat on either side of her lover's hips. She sits on his lap with her legs spread wide for penetration (and for a great view for him!), and rests her own weight on her hands, which are behind her and grasping his ankles or shins. She does most of the work here, lifting herself up and down on his penis.

WHERE TO DO IT

The bed is the most comfortable place to do the Seesaw sex position, but any wide open space (like the floor) will also do.

PROPS YOU'LL NEED

None.

DIFFICULTY LEVEL ★☆☆☆☆

HER O-METER ★★★☆☆

For the Seesaw sex position to truly be effective, she must be totally and completely comfortable with her partner. Since she is open for him to see every inch of her in this sex position, she's got to be comfortable with herself as well. Confident girls will like this sex position because it gives their lovers such pleasure to see them spread out. She'll also enjoy the intimacy of being able to look him in the eye as they both experience orgasm.

HIS O-METER ★★★★★

He's comfortable in the Seesaw sex position, and he really enjoys it because he can simply sit back, relax, and watch as she grinds, rotates, and thrusts all over him. With her legs spread open, he can see everything that is happening, and that kind of visual stimulation is exactly what he needs to take a hot sex position to the next level.

MAKE IT HOTTER . . .

The more she gets into the show for him, the better this position will be!

SEXY CHALLENGE:

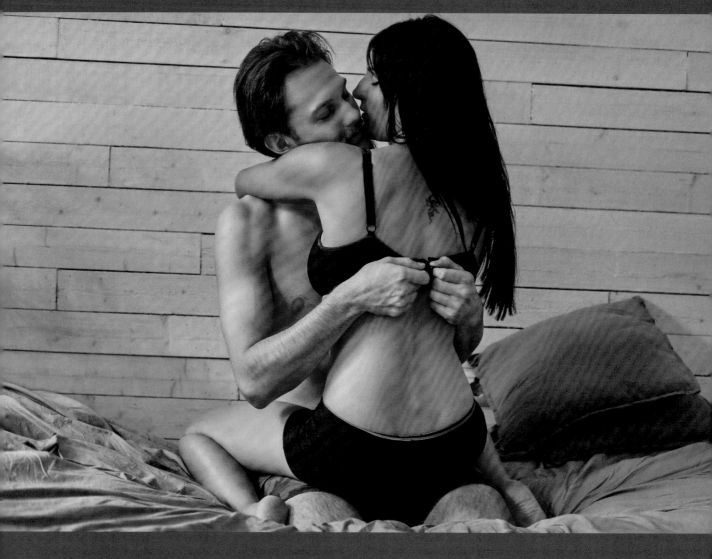

WITHIN THE SACRED GARDEN

There is a power in just being together as one! This power can be felt and enjoyed without the aggressive actions we most often associate with sexual activity. The movement, the thrusting, and the repetition are amazing and powerful, but this challenge is to really feel what it is like to be inside your partner, not the friction that is going to bring about orgasm. The sitting position can allow us to just be one with each other for a time period, allowing us to slowly bring ourselves to a place of arousal that allows you to stop and smell every rose along the way; to truly enjoy the process of sexual arousal and excitement.

Sensations are going to be intense in this Sexy Challenge. Not only because of the physical sensations, but also because of the energetic and emotional sensations created by being locked together. Most of the time during sex, we feel our own pleasure and we might experience the pleasure of our partner as they climax. But what does it truly feel like to be inside their body of have them inside you? Can you feel what they feel? Do your senses connect? Sitting positions allow you to experience all these things within the sacred garden of togetherness.

This Sexy Challenge is not meant to be rushed, so if you are in a hurry, save this one for another day. This challenge will often benefit the ladies more than the men in a physical nature. However, in a mindful state, it will connect partners in a deeper and more meaningful way. Now, guys, don't worry; you are going to experience the pleasure you desire, but you might have to be a little patient. The object of this challenge is to be one with your partner, to truly connect.

Positions such as the Lotus or Pretzel are perfect for this experience, as we start by just getting inside our partner or allowing our partners energy to flow inside us. Once we are connected as one, we can begin to completely experience the sensations, and see how they affect us as we are connected to our partner in this sacred garden. Try breathing together to enhance the connection. Once connected, take turns just lightly running your hands down your partner's back. See if you can feel the excitement they are feeling when you touch them. Sometimes you will feel spasms within the genitals, which are obvious. If the penis jumps while in the vagina, both partners will feel that, or if the vagina tightens, the same physical feeling happens. We want to go much deeper than just the physically obvious feelings, though.

See if running your hands lightly down your partner's back might give you the goosebumps or chills. Close your eyes, and see if you feel the sensation of a hand lightly running down your back while you are doing it to your partner. But don't stop there; start to see what other sensations you can perform on your partner and how they affect your body while you are locked together. See what passionate kissing feels like in this connection, or slap your partner on the ass, or play with their nipples hard or softly. Then have your partner touch you and see if they get any sensations of these experiences. Try closing your eyes while this is going on, and then try gazing deeply into your partner's eyes while this is going on. Any crazy thing you want to try, go for it. You might just be amazed at what you can feel through your partner's body.

Don't stop there; try to put some outside influences into this sexual experiment. Maybe get some mirrors and place them around, so you can see all the angles as you are touching your partner. Try out different locations in your house—there could be a drastic difference in the sensations by moving out of the bedroom and into the living room. You might even branch out to a neutral place, such as a hotel. You can make it more interesting by trying it in the bathtub or shower. You can also add different types of music playing in the background. Try out hot and cold items on each other, like ice cubes, heating pads, and wax, which can all be super exciting and transferable with this amazing energy. Be creative with this, and just open yourself up to see what experiences you receive. You might not have any, or you might have something amazing.

One word of caution, however: don't "expect" any sensations! Allow them to come into you naturally. Trying to force them will put up walls that might make it impossible for your connected sensations to come through. One time this might work amazingly for you, and the next, you might not get anything; it just depends on all the situations. Also, if you don't feel anything, don't think your partner is the wrong person for you. Have fun with this, and accept what you get out of it. If nothing else, you are going to have a great time connecting with the person you are with. Then, after you get down with the experience of the Sacred Garden, you can switch gears and get as wild and crazy as you want.

CHAPTER 7: STANDING SEX POSITIONS

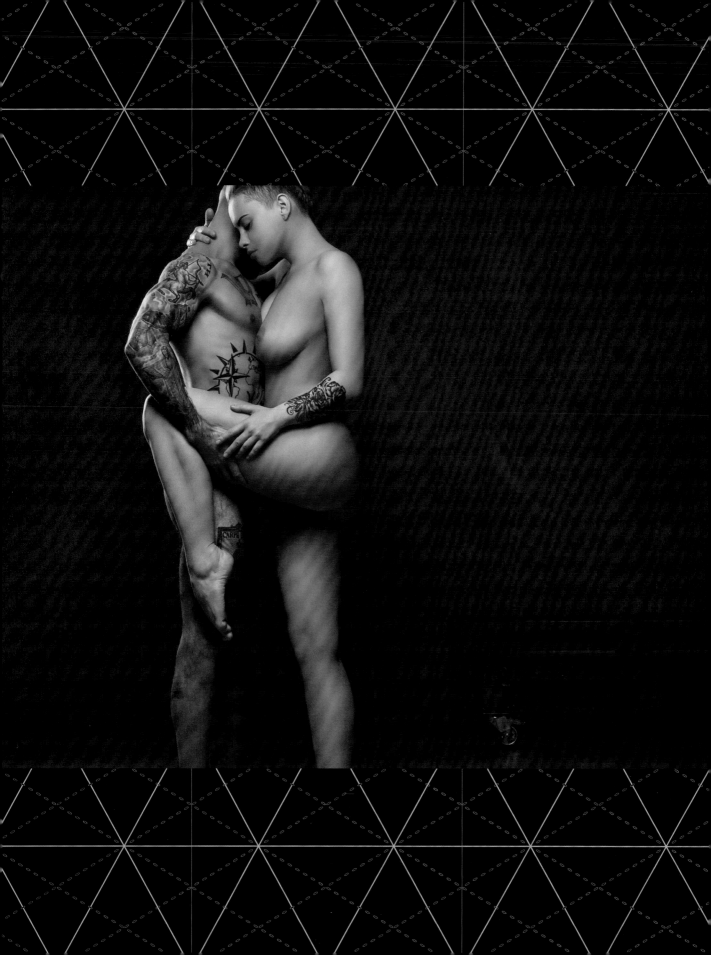

DANCER

Experience incredibly hot, "I need you right now," sex with the Dancer sex position! It can be a bit difficult to master if you're not used to standing sex positions, but if you can get aligned properly, it's a super-hot, yet intimate, sex position to try. He feels totally in control here!

HOW TO DO IT

Both partners stand facing each other, (like regular Missionary, only upright), and the female lifts either leg, causing her knee to bend at a ninety-degree angle. This makes it easier for the male partner to thrust, while gripping her thigh or buttocks for leverage. This sex position is super sexy because it's often thought of as the "I need you now" sex position. It's as if neither of you wants to find somewhere to have sex, take your clothes off, and lie down—you want to do it right here, right now.

WHERE TO DO IT

Dancer can be done anywhere you can stand!

PROPS YOU'LL NEED

A wall or chair if you're not particularly strong or don't have good balance. Leaning up against the wall can make this position more stable.

DIFFICULTY LEVEL ★★★☆☆

HER O-METER ★★★☆☆

Standing sex is hot. It's primal, and conveys that he wants her now and can't wait. Women love to be wanted, craved, and desired. If he wants her so badly that he can't wait to have sex until he gets her to the bedroom, she'll be totally into it.

HIS O-METER ★★★★☆

He loves standing sex just as much. He loves feeling dominant and in control. This sex position makes him feel totally in control and very much like a man.

MAKE IT HOTTER . . .

This sex position is awesome for public sex because you can do it pretty much anywhere. It's quick, it's dirty, and it's totally hot. Guys, make it even hotter by throwing your girl up against a wall (firm, but not too hard—you just want to take her by surprise). Grab her leg and hitch it up around your hips. Make it clear that you want her now, right now.

BALLERINA

The Ballerina sex position is a popular standing sex position that is an excellent choice for very flexible women! Women who aren't as flexible may find this position difficult to get into and stay in though, so if you can't hike your leg up that far, consider another position, or practice stretching until you can comfortably get into the Ballerina.

HOW TO DO IT

In the Ballerina sex position, both partners are standing facing each other. The female partner raises one of her legs all the way up, resting her ankle on her lover's shoulder. Yes, she has to be incredibly flexible to do this! He holds on to her leg with one hand and her hip with the other, and is responsible for the majority of the thrusting movement.

Less flexible women can simply wrap one leg around her lover's waist (a.k.a. the Dancer sex position).

WHERE TO DO IT

Standing sex positions are awesome to do in tight spaces, like when you want a quickie in the closet at a party, or are at home and don't want the kids to catch you.

PROPS YOU'LL NEED

None.

DIFFICULTY LEVEL ★★★★★

HER O-METER ★☆☆☆☆

She's going to be more concerned about stretching comfortably and staying upright in the Ballerina sex position, so she's not terribly into getting an orgasm out of it. But if she does get into it, the penetration is deep enough to elicit G-spot stimulation and possible orgasms!

HIS O-METER ★★★★☆

He totally digs her leg raised like this, and if she can do the Ballerina sex position, he'll be convinced his sex life is awesome. Guys tend to like more exotic sex positions (you know, the ones where the woman is folded up like a pretzel in a near impossible configuration), so this is high up on his "I just want to try this" list.

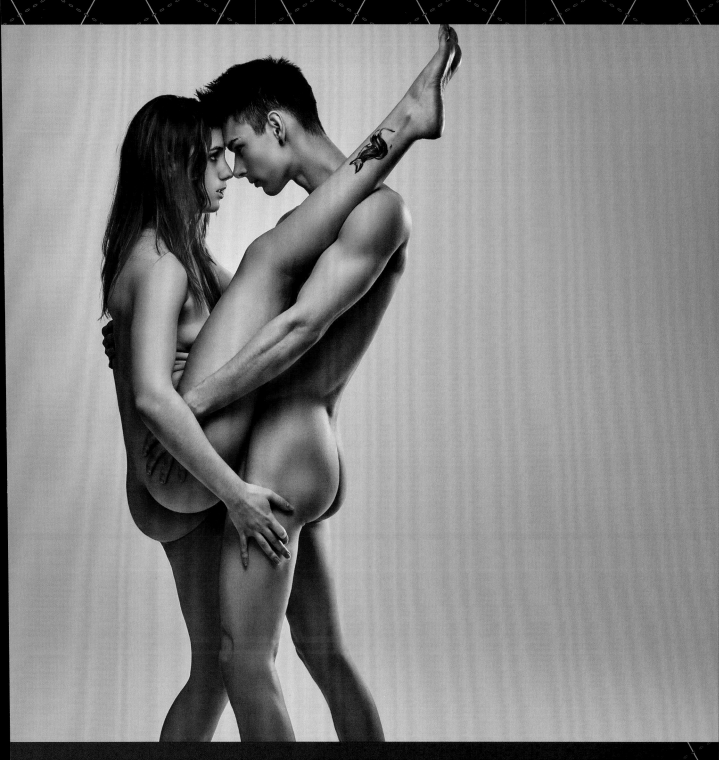

MAKE IT HOTTER . . .

Try the Ballerina sex position outside the house. Slip into a public bathroom stall and get it on there (just don't touch anything!), or in a dressing room at the department store.

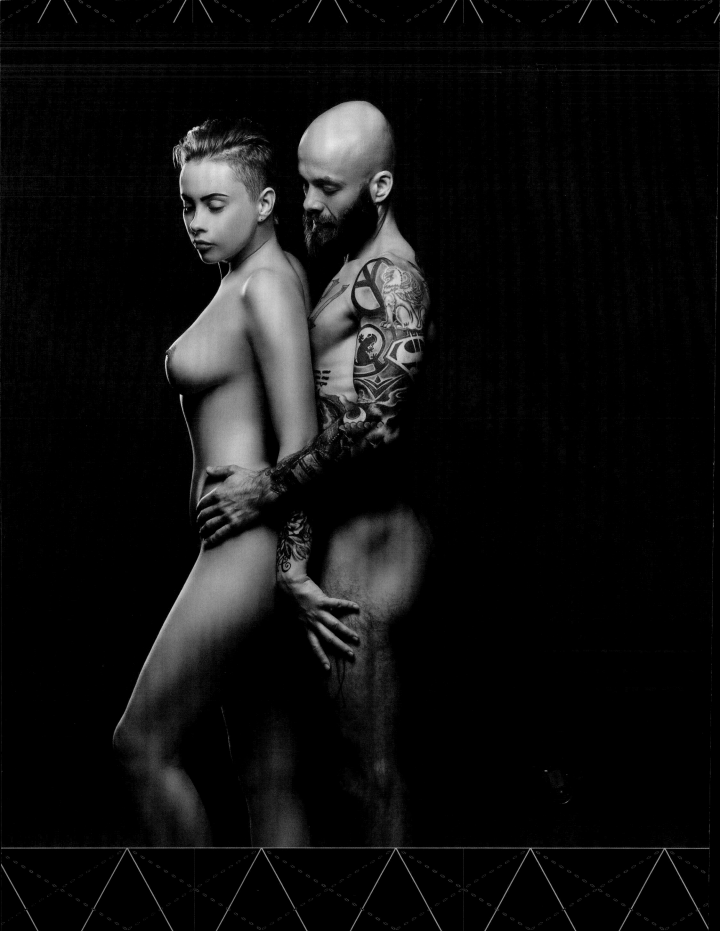

BODYGUARD

This is a sex position in which good thrusting can be difficult to achieve (especially if she's short), but if you can get lined up properly, the Bodyguard can be extremely intimate and satisfying. He can touch her anywhere, kiss her neck, and whisper dirty things in her ear!

HOW TO DO IT

The Bodyguard is a standing, rear-entry sex position that isn't too hard to actually get into, but it's a little difficult and awkward to keep up during thrusting. Height differences between partners can make it a little more challenging, but it's certainly not impossible. In this sex position, both partners stand, with the female partner resting her back against her lover's chest. He enters her from behind, and both partners slightly bend their knees to facilitate thrusting. It may take a few minutes to get in sync, but this position can be super intimate. It's important for the female partner to arch her back, or else he may keep "slipping out."

WHERE TO DO IT

The shower, closet, or anywhere else you can stand are all great options. Ideally the Bodyguard is performed in front of a mirror for the visual enjoyment of both partners.

PROPS YOU'LL NEED

If the partners vary greatly in height, add a footstool (or stairs) to help even things out. This will better line up the partners' genitals for ease of thrusting.

DIFFICULTY LEVEL ★★★★☆

HER O-METER ★☆☆☆☆

The Bodyguard isn't a favorite among women, unless their partners have longer penises. A smaller penis doesn't penetrate as far in this position, and can leave a woman wanting more. (Men with smaller penises who want to engage in rear entry sex are better off using the Doggy Style (see page 244) or Standing Doggy Style (see page 176) sex positions, as they encourage deeper penetration.) He can make the Bodyguard better for her by reaching his hands around to her front to fondle her breasts, nipples, and clitoris.

HIS O-METER ★★★☆☆

He likes this position fairly well, but it's a little lackluster for him unless you're doing it in front of a mirror (which is a great idea, by the way). Men need visual stimulation to really enjoy sex, and without a mirror, there's not much for him to look at here. If he's a breast man, he will particularly like it when she arches her back and pushes her breasts up and out for him to fondle.

MAKE IT HOTTER...

This is a great sex position to use in the shower, especially if you have a smaller shower stall. Since you can't really lie down in a lot of showers, the Bodyguard is a great way to still have wet and wild sex in the bathroom! Just make sure to use a good-quality lube, since water washes away bodily secretions.

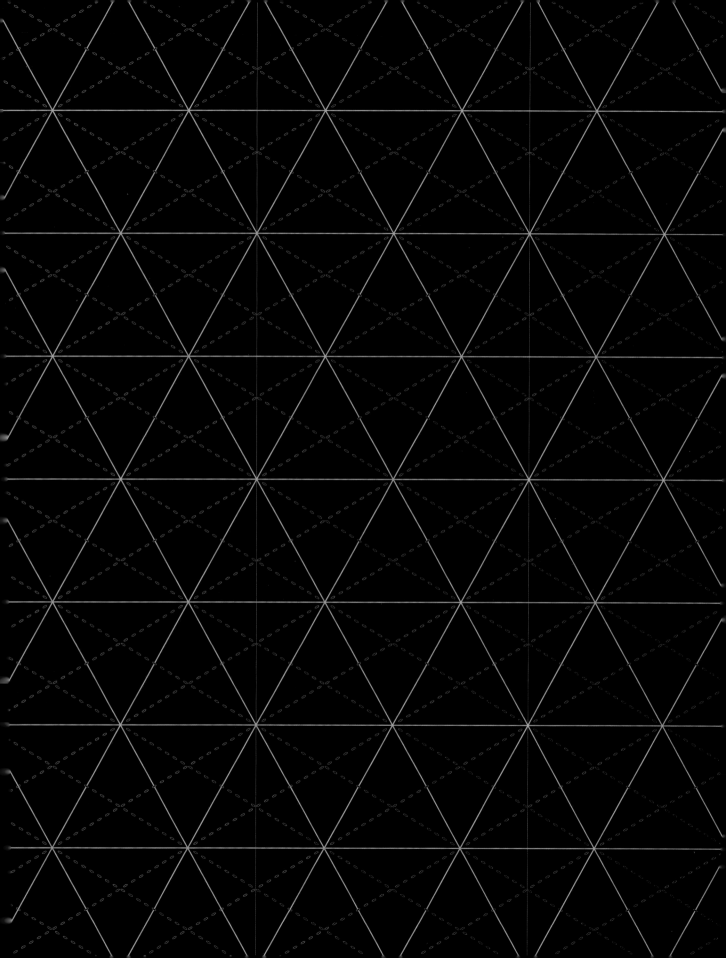

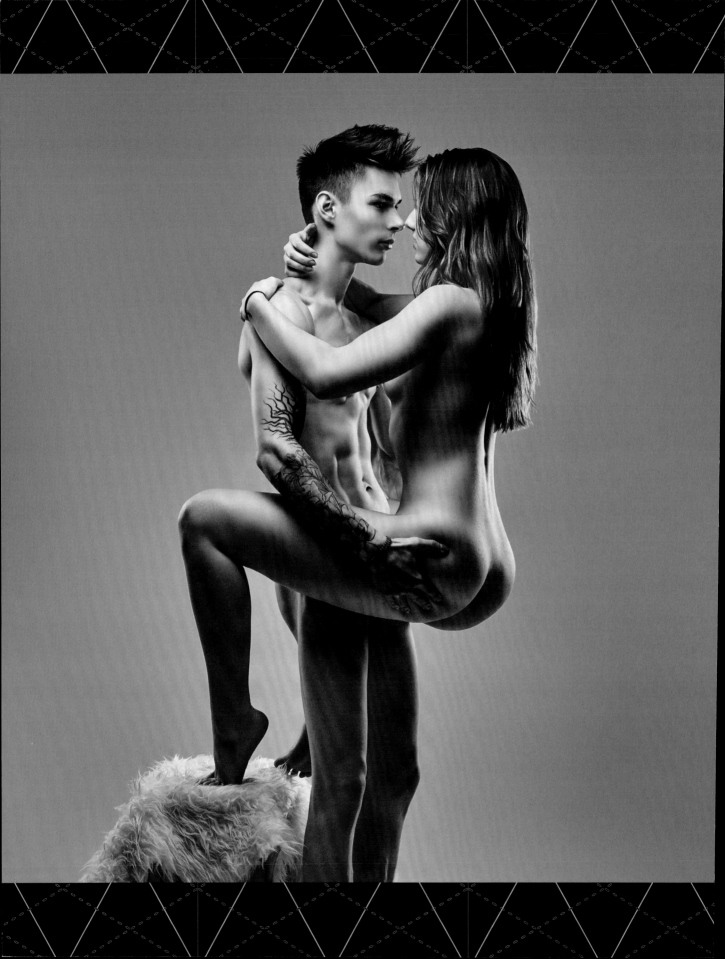

PISTON

The Piston sex position is a great standing position for athletic couples, and allows super-deep and exotic penetration. It's definitely a must try!

HOW TO DO IT

The male partner stands with his back to a chair or sofa, facing his female partner. He lifts her onto his penis (which is no small accomplishment), and she rests her feet on the surface behind him, using the leverage to help with the thrusting movements. The Piston sex position isn't easy to do for most couples, because it requires plenty of arm strength on his part to hold almost her entire weight, and lots of leg strength on her part.

WHERE TO DO IT

The piston can be done anywhere in the house where you have a surface she can rest her feet on.

PROPS YOU'LL NEED

None.

DIFFICULTY LEVEL ★★★★★

HER O-METER ★★★☆☆

Although the Piston sex position may require her to have substantial leg strength, it's worth it for all of the clitoral friction she gets. With as much effort as she is putting into the thrusting, it may be difficult for her to focus on building an orgasm, but if she's very athletic, it won't bother her a bit, and she can truly enjoy what this awesome sex position has to offer!

HIS O-METER ★★★☆☆

He likes holding her up and thrusting deeply into her, although the Piston sex position can get quite tiring for him. If he's very fit, he'll be able to keep it up for a little while, but not necessarily long enough for both him and her to have an orgasm. This is a fun sex position to try for a little while before moving on to something more comfortable.

MAKE IT HOTTER . . .

Both partners are going to be pretty occupied with supporting their weight and getting the movement down pat, so focus more on that than what you can do to "spice" this sex position up. The Piston sex position is pretty hot in and of itself!

PRISON GUARD

The Prison Guard sex position is a wonderfully submissive position for the woman that allows for both vaginal rear entry intercourse and anal sex.

HOW TO DO IT

The Prison Guard sex position is a fairly easy position to get into, since both partners are standing. The female partner is standing up against her man, with her back to him, and is bent over almost as far as she can go. She will bring her hands up behind her back for her partner to grasp and hold onto as he thrusts, mimicking "handcuffs" and lending the Prison Guard sex position its name.

WHERE TO DO IT

Standing sex positions are exceptionally versatile when it comes to where you can do them. You can do them in the middle of the living room, or in tighter quarters like the bathroom or even a closet. You can do the Prison Guard sex position almost anywhere you can stand!

PROPS YOU'LL NEED

None.

DIFFICULTY LEVEL ★☆☆☆☆

HER O-METER ★★★☆☆

If she enjoys being very submissive, she's going to love the Prison Guard sex position. She'll also like it if she enjoys lots (and lots!) of the intense sensations that deep penetration gives. However, it's not going to be her favorite if she can only get off with more clitoral stimulation, since this sex position doesn't afford any clitoral friction at all.

HIS O-METER ★★★★★

He really enjoys the Prison Guard sex position because it allows him complete control over his partner! She is deeply submitting to him, and not only does he get to bind her wrists with his hands, he gets to watch the action as he thrusts. If he enjoys being dominant, this is likely to be one of his favorite sex positions.

MAKE IT HOTTER . . .

The Prison Guard sex position can be used for really kinky, naughty anal sex, but only if both partners are no strangers to anal play. This is not an anal sex position for beginners; however, it can be really hot for lovers who have done anal a few times before.

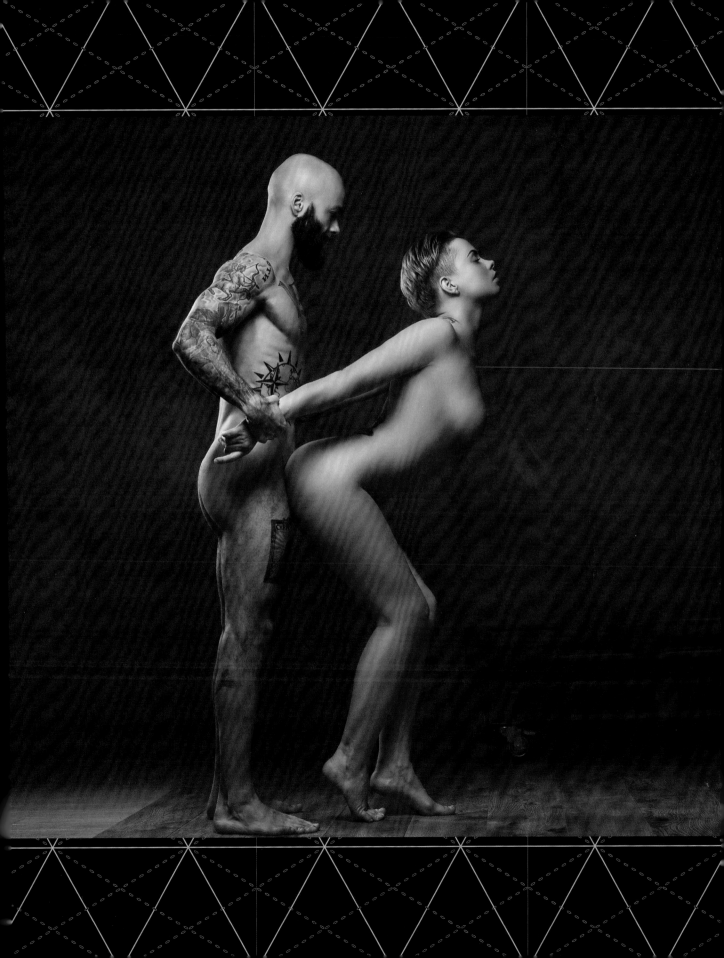

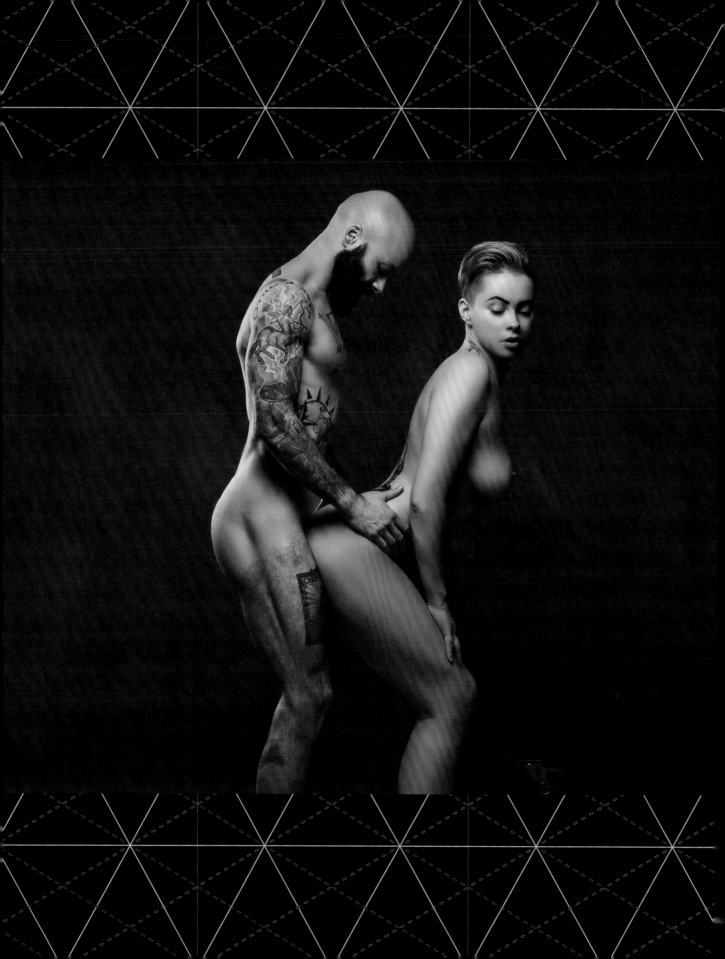

SQUAT

The Squat is a challenging standing position that requires lots of balance on the female partner's part. It's fun to try if you can do it!

HOW TO DO IT

For the male partner, the Squat sex position is particularly simple, because all he's doing is standing in front of his partner, who is facing away from him. She stands on an ottoman or stool (a chair is likely going to be too high), and squats down, bringing her buttocks close to her lover's groin. He holds on to her hips as he thrusts. The Squat sex position is great for both rear-entry and anal sex!

WHERE TO DO IT

As with almost all standing sex positions, the Squat is very versatile in terms of where it can be performed. You may want to do it at home, where you have access to different things for her to stand on (this will help you achieve a comfortable height), but it can be done anywhere you can stand.

PROPS YOU'LL NEED

None.

DIFFICULTY LEVEL ★★★☆☆

HER O-METER ★☆☆☆☆

The Squat sex position is more difficult for her than it is pleasurable. She may dig the deep penetration, but she may feel like she's going to fall off the stool or ottoman with the thrusting. It's also going to be very easy for her to get leg cramps in this position, even if she's quite athletic.

HIS O-METER ★★★★☆

He totally loves the Squat sex position because it's easy for him to do and he gets to watch all the action. If he likes butts, he's really going to enjoy caressing, squeezing, and playing with her buttocks. He may be disappointed if she can't keep this sex position up for long, but it's definitely one that is difficult for her to stay in for any significant period of time.

MAKE IT HOTTER...

If both partners are into anal play, he can easily use his hands, fingers, or a sex toy to give her anal stimulation during intercourse.

STANDING DOGGY STYLE

Standing Doggy Style is easier on the knees than traditional Doggy Style, and still provides the same perks for both female and male partners. This is another fun, "animal-style" sex position, because all you have to do for a quickie is pull your pants and underwear down!

HOW TO DO IT

Standing Doggy Style is a little bit easier on the knees than traditional Doggy Style, mainly because both partners are standing up. This does require some kind of prop, like a chair, sofa, or bed, but it's relatively simple to do. While standing, the female partner bends at the waist and places the palms of her hands on the chosen prop. The male partner enters her from behind, standing the entire time.

WHERE TO DO IT

Standing Doggy can be done anywhere that she has room to bend over and support herself with her hands. Try the bed, sofa, stairs, and the hood of the car. Just use your imagination!

PROPS YOU'LL NEED

A chair, sofa, or bed to lean on.

DIFFICULTY LEVEL ★☆☆☆☆

HER O-METER ★★★☆☆

Like traditional Doggy Style, this position is fairly good for G-spot penetration. It's much more difficult for her to reach her clitoris, however, because she's supporting the majority of her weight with her hands. She'll enjoy this position more if he reaches down and stimulates her clitoris.

HIS O-METER ★★★★☆

Standing Doggy Style provides as good a view as traditional Doggy Style, and men really dig the idea of the backdoor action, even if they're not actually getting to go in the "back door."

MAKE IT HOTTER . . .

Standing Doggy Style is another one of those "got to have it now" sex positions. Both partners can drop their drawers and go at it pretty much anytime, anywhere. It's incredibly hot to want your partner so bad that you really can't even take the time to undress all the way.

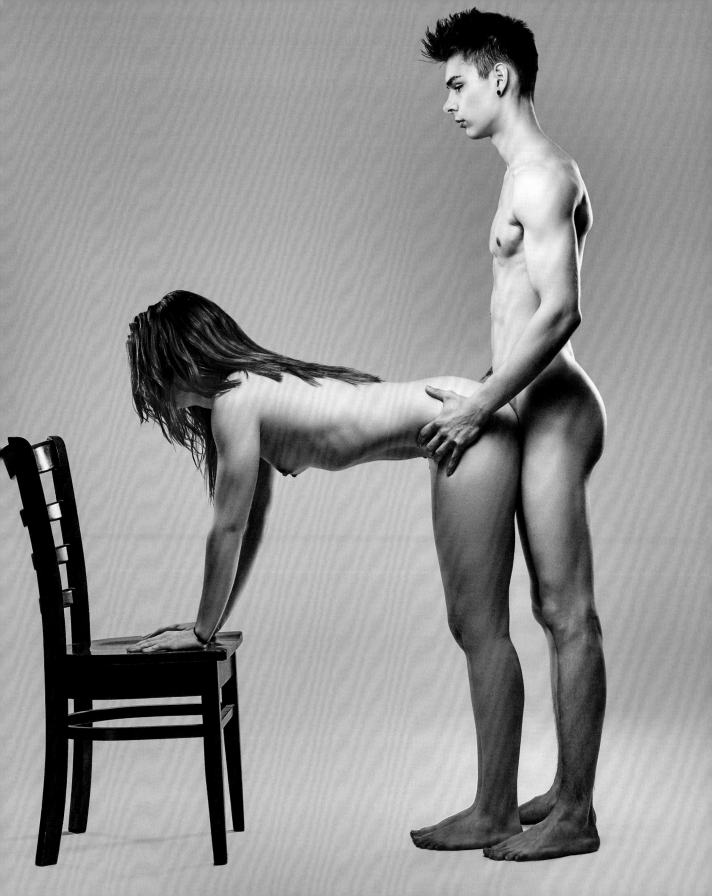

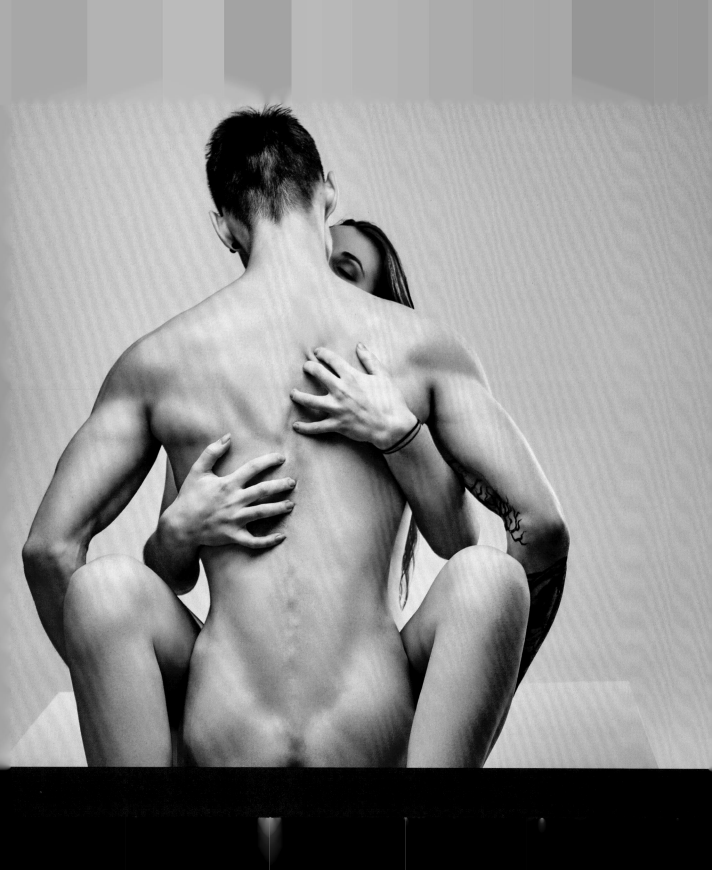

KINGS AND QUEENS— PUTTING YOUR LOVE ON A PEDESTAL

Standing sex positions are not the easiest sex positions, that is for sure. They require stamina and other elements, such as height and position of the genitals on the body, to make it work effectively. Even with that, standing sex positions help couples mix things up in an amazing fashion. Standing sex is a great workout for both partners, and afterwards you can usually feel the burn in your legs, just as you would from leg day at the gym. It can also help with some areas of sexual problems, such as premature ejaculation, as it isn't as easy to thrust for the male in most of these positions. With all that being said, there is still an excitement around the standing sex positions; it is a position of royalty, designated for the kings and queens to put their love on a pedestal.

Think of all the great sculptures of the past standing on their pedestals in the museums. We are amazed at their beauty and detail. We want to do the same for your standing sex. As was mentioned earlier, standing sex is reserved for royalty, and we want you to approach it that way. You both are the King and Queen of your kingdom and your sex should be honored as such. Standing sex helps you keep the royal sheets clean, as well as allowing both partners to see their naked King or Queen in a different light during their lovemaking. These positions also help your royal sex rise above normal and typical sex where you are laying down.

The first thing you have to do to become the King and Queen of standing sex is to get into the feeling that you are royalty. Think of your body as a divine instrument, with the purpose to bring about amazing things to your kingdom. Address your body parts as royalty. You now have the Royal Penis upon your body, and the Royal Sacred Space for the Royal Penis is in the Imperial Vagina. Have fun creating royal names for all your body parts, such as the Immaculate Breasts, the Stately Buttocks, etc. Have fun with this, because it can be a real turn on. Once you assume the role of royalty, you might just find that alone will help ramp up the energy of the illustrious sex you are about to have.

The next thing you need to do is to find a wrap to cover the royal body. It can be a robe, a blanket, or even a bath sheet. This is for when it comes time to stand in front of your King or Queen, and present your royal body to them by removing the royal covering. When you do this, think of the posture of a king and queen: no slouching, just throw your shoulders back and let your royalty shine. Stride up to your partner, and place yourself in front of him/her, then correct your posture and simply let your wrap drop to the floor. Present your royal body to your lover, and let them gander upon your exquisite body. Be proud of your body. I know that is difficult for a lot of people. If this is difficult for you, you can do several things such, as dim the lights or turn them out completely, and maybe have a flameless candle burning in the room. Just a hint of light in the room will allow your king or queen to see your body, but will hide some of the areas you might be uncomfortable about.

Once all royal members have presented their naked royal bodies to each other, the royal couple should move closer, and just barely let their bodies touch, allowing a light blast of energy to flow through each other. Feel the hardened nipples of the Queen gently scrape across the King's chest; feel the King's penis lightly touch the inner thigh of the Queen. Then pull each other close and let the energy begin flowing with a kiss. Be ready for the tidal wave of excitement to run through your body. You might even hear the cheers of the Kingdom as the royal lovemaking is about to begin. One of you might even announce it in a royal manner: "The Royal Screwing is about to Begin!". At this point, you both can move in even closer to prepare for standing sex. I suggest trying the Dancer and/or the Standing Doggy Style positions in this chapter, as they might seem a little more royal than the Prison Guard position.

During your standing sex experiences, keep your mind focused on being royalty. This about how the energy of your sexual experience will benefit your kingdom. Think about how exciting it is to be sharing your royal body with another body of royalty. Imagine the power that comes to your kingdom from the amazing sexual experience. Allow the waves of pleasure to splash over and over your body, until your bodies seem to be floating above the ground as you near the point of climactic bliss. Once that moment happens, and both of you return to having your feet down upon your king-dom, you need to honor your celebration of orgasmic energy. Step back from each other and either bow or curtsy to your partner as a sign of a job well done for both of you.

At this point, it is important for the royal couples to become clean. So, we suggest moving the royal party to the shower, and enjoying the blissful sensation of the cleans-ing waters of your Kingdom. Now, as royalty, it is important that you understand that you would have someone to help bathe you. Take turns washing each other's royal bodies, and, if things go well, you might be performing another act of sexual royalty in the shower. Yes, it is good to be the King and Queen.

To make this experience even more powerful, let's add some bonus suggestions. Number one, if you have a party store in your town, you could go there and pick up some fun props, such as crowns, robes, and even royal jewelry. Also, if the Queen doesn't usually climax through vaginal intercourse, then you might need to seek out Merlin's magic wand (a vibrator) to help the Queen reach her royal place. Items such as body jewelry, cock rings, and even body oils, can be used to rub each other down first and can heighten the experience. I would also suggest a feast of food before or after the event: grapes, strawberries, cheese, and other finger foods that you could sexy challenge: kings and queens—putting your love on a pedestal   181

feed to your royal partner. Even a little wine poured into a goblet would be a nice touch to bring this Sexy Challenge full circle.

The famous line "My Kingdom for a Horse" will now be changed to "Forget the Horse; Let's Screw for the Kingdom."

CHAPTER 8: SIDE-BY-SIDE SEX POSITIONS

CRAZY STARFISH

For a super exotic sex position that you can add to your "we tried" list, the Crazy Starfish is fun, yet very challenging, for both partners.

HOW TO DO IT

Both partners will lie on their sides facing the same way, but head to toe with each other. The female partner will lower herself onto him with her legs wrapped around his waist, and he will in turn wrap his own legs around her waist. He can brace his hands on her thighs to help facilitate thrusting, and she can support her weight with her arms behind her.

WHERE TO DO IT

The bed is the best place for this one—this one requires a good deal of space. The floor works too, but carpet burns hurt! This is definitely not one you can do in a narrow space like the sofa or the back seat of a car. Too many limbs everywhere!

PROPS YOU'LL NEED

None.

DIFFICULTY LEVEL ★★★☆

HER O-METER ★★★☆☆

She doesn't have a whole lot of clitoral contact here in the Crazy Starfish, but the G-spot stimulation helps make up for it.

HIS O-METER ★★★★☆

He absolutely loves the view he gets in the Crazy Starfish, and he loves to watch the action. Bonus points for the "exotic" factor here! The only caveat for him is that his penis is bent slightly at an awkward angle, but it's likely not enough for him to be uncomfortable.

MAKE IT HOTTER . . .

He can make the Crazy Starfish way hotter for her by using his hands or a sex toy to play with her clitoris. She is at a perfect angle for him to do this, so he really should do something so that both partners can get off! If she wants to give him something even more to look at, she can, of course, take matters into her own hands.

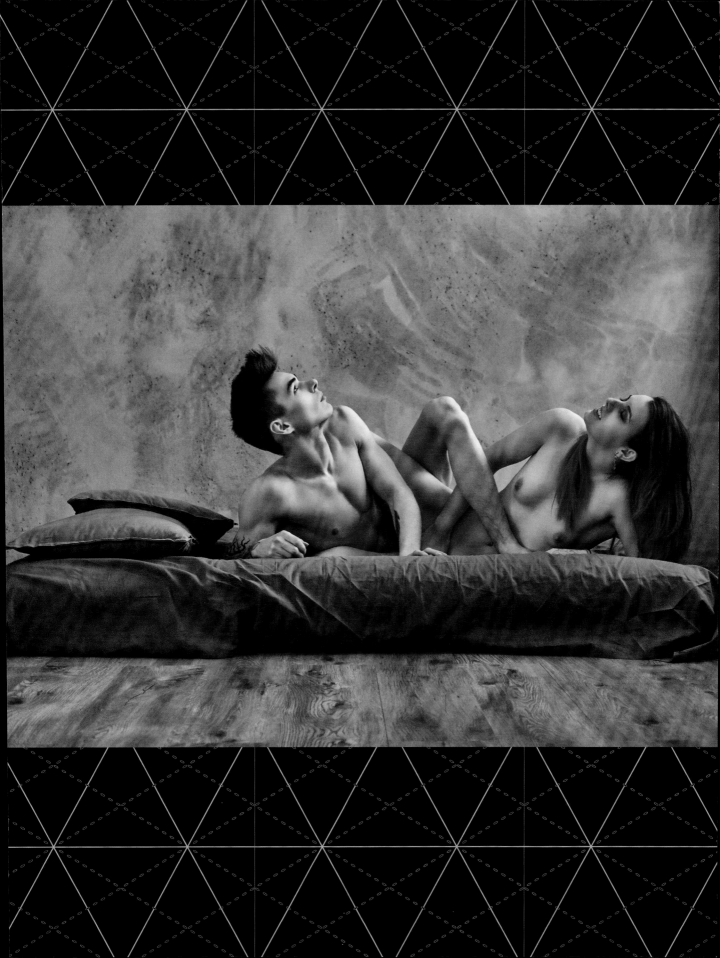

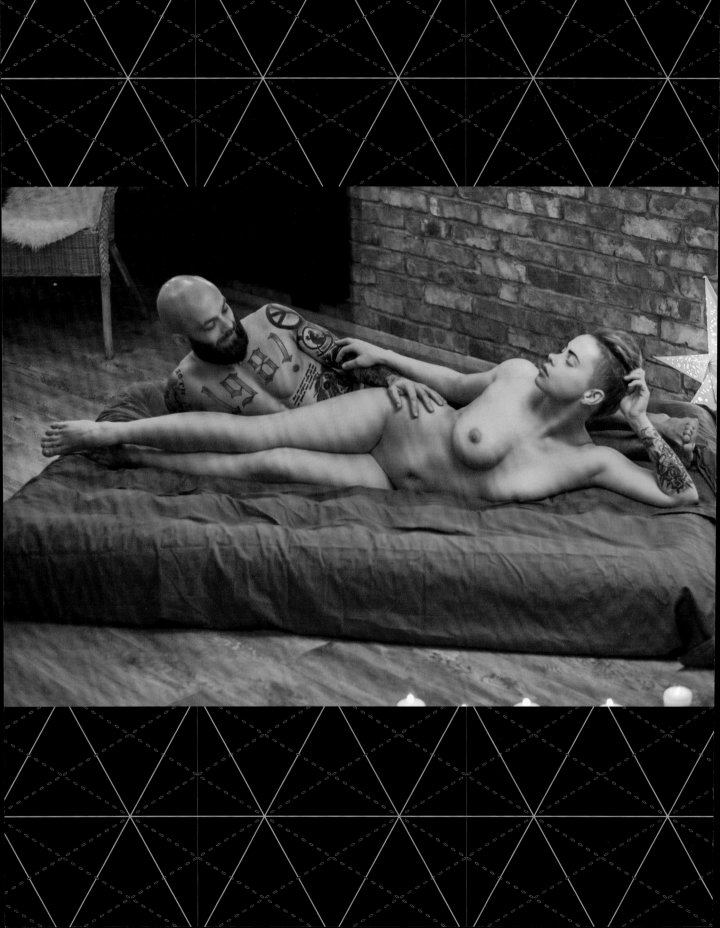

INVERTED SPOON

The Inverted Spoon is a unique position for side-by-side fun that is a bit kinkier than traditional spooning. It's exotic, yet still intimate!

HOW TO DO IT

The male partner lies down on his side on a flat surface, and his partner lies on her side facing away from him, with her back to him, and with her head to his feet and her feet to his head. He can place his hands on her thighs or hips to help him thrust. This one will work a little better for most couples if they both bend at the waist just a bit. This makes for a better angle of penetration. Otherwise his penis can be at an uncomfortable angle.

WHERE TO DO IT

The Inverted Spoon requires a great deal of space length wise, since both partners are completely stretched out. The bed is perfect for this, although the floor will work as well. If you have a futon or pull-out couch, you can use that for a change in venue.

PROPS YOU'LL NEED

None.

DIFFICULTY LEVEL ★☆☆☆☆

HER O-METER ★★★☆☆

She likes the Inverted Spoon because it's easy for her lover to reach around and fondle her clitoris, or she can do it herself. She can also fondle her nipples during lovemaking, and he can, too, if he is able to reach.

HIS O-METER ★★★☆☆

"Butt guys" will love this sex position! It's a kinky twist on traditional spooning and is definitely one he will want to try. He likes the view and the feel of her butt grinding up against him.

MAKE IT HOTTER . . .

She can raise one leg up to allow her lover to get a really nice view, although she'll need to be pretty self-confident to do this, because everything will be on display! However, this move will take the "hot" factor up a few notches. The Inverted Spoon can also be used for anal sex if both partners enjoy a little backdoor action from time to time.

LINGUINI

The Linguini sex position is great for deep penetration and for letting yourself go in the moment.

HOW TO DO IT

The female partner lies on her side with a pillow under her head for extra support. While she lounges, the male partner kneels directly behind her butt and pushes one of his knees between her legs for insertion. The trick to this position is for the female partner to be relaxed and keep her limbs loose, so that the male partner can penetrate her deeply.

WHERE TO DO IT

The Linguini sex position is best performed in the bed. While the floor will work, the bed is certainly the most comfortable option. If you do decide to do it on the floor, make sure you have plenty of blankets and pillows. A soft surface is a must!

PROPS YOU'LL NEED

Blankets and pillows will make sure she is relaxed and comfortable.

DIFFICULTY LEVEL ★★★☆☆

HER O-METER ★★★★☆

She likes the Linguini sex position because she can just sit back and enjoy the ride. That, coupled with the unique angle of G-spot stimulation, can make the Linguini sex position extremely orgasmic for her!

HIS O-METER ★★★★☆

This side-by-side position causes her thighs to be curved at an angle which gives him deeper access. He'll love to hear her moan as he stimulates her G-spot with ease.

MAKE IT HOTTER . . .

While staying relaxed is important for the Linguini, it is critical for her to show him that she's enjoying herself, as this position can tend to make her look bored if she's not actively showing her joy.

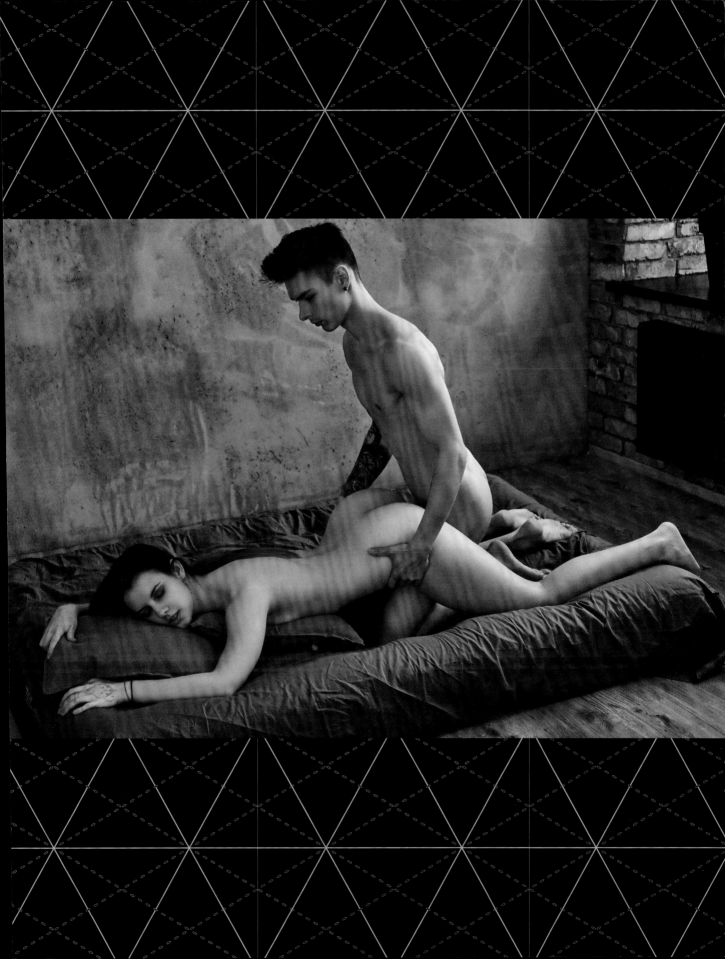

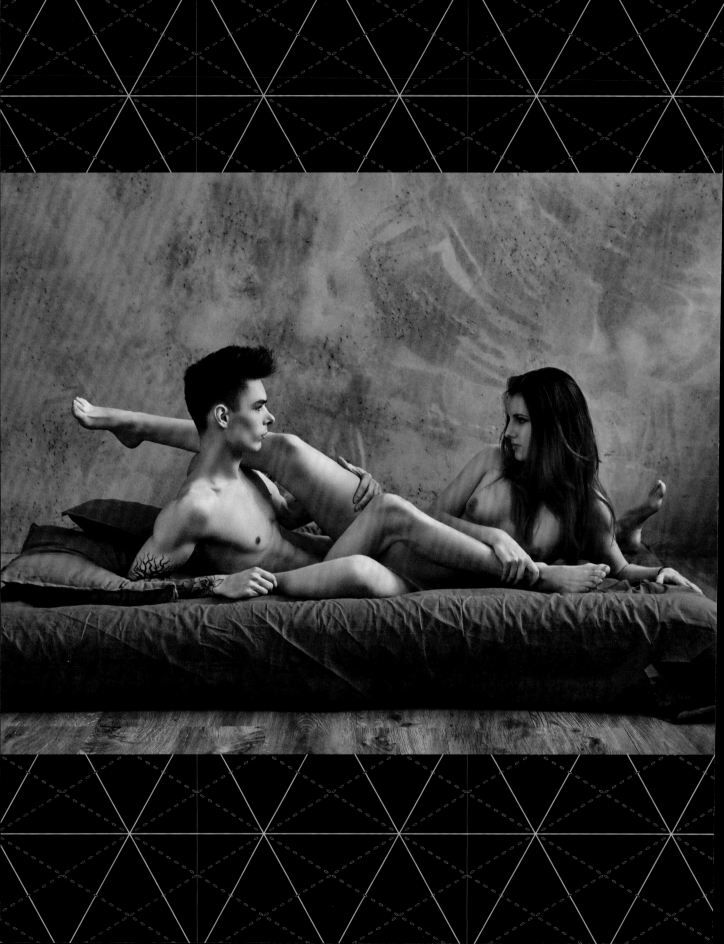

SCISSORS

The Scissors is an exotic sex position that is easy to do, and is great to use when others won't work, like during pregnancy.

HOW TO DO IT

The male partner lies on his side on a bed, and lifts one of his legs so that his legs are wide open. His partner lies on her back or side, perpendicular to him, straddling the leg that he has lifted so her groin is pressed against his and he is able to penetrate her. He can grasp one of her legs, and she can support her weight on her arms to help with thrusting.

WHERE TO DO IT

The Scissors sex position requires so much space that you're better off doing it in the bed. While the floor will work, the bed is certainly the most comfortable option. If you do decide to do it on the floor, make sure you have plenty of blankets and pillows! It's also a fun sex position to do outdoors on a picnic blanket if you have enough privacy!

PROPS YOU'LL NEED

Add some pillows for extra support here and there.

DIFFICULTY LEVEL ★★★☆☆

HER O-METER ★★★★☆

She likes the Scissors position because it's exceptionally easy for her to get clitoral stimulation. She can grind her clitoris up against his thigh, and with some lube, it can feel absolutely fantastic. That, coupled with the unique angle of G-spot stimulation, can make the Scissors position extremely orgasmic for her! Although this is an "exotic" sex position, it actually works quite well during pregnancy, when a woman isn't able to lie flat on her back in the later stages of pregnancy, and can't be on top when she gets bigger.

HIS O-METER ★★★★☆

He likes being able to watch her get off in this position, and the angle of penetration makes sex feel different and new for him, too. This is a great position to use if you're looking for something fairly exotic, but also fairly easy!

MAKE IT HOTTER . . .

This is a great position for her to reach down and stimulate her clitoris during sex, either with her fingers or a good clitoral vibrator.

SPOONING

As far as romantic and intimate sex positions go, Spooning is really where it's at. Much like spooning when sleeping or cuddling, this sex position provides full body contact and plenty of opportunities for touching, hugging, kissing, and whispering in each other's ears.

HOW TO DO IT

This is a wonderfully intimate sex position that will give both partners a sense of emotional connection. While both partners are lying on their sides, he enters her from behind, with his chest resting up against her back. This is very much like the "spooning" position that many couples use while sleeping, which makes this sex position so comforting and sensual.

WHERE TO DO IT

The Spooning sex position works well anywhere you can snuggle, such as on the sofa while watching a movie and, of course, in the bed.

PROPS YOU'LL NEED

None.

DIFFICULTY LEVEL ★☆☆☆☆

HER O-METER ★★★☆☆

She will really enjoy the intimacy of this sex position. It feels very much like cuddling to her, which is right up her alley. The penetration might not be as deep as other sex positions. However, he can make up for this by reaching around and stroking her skin with his hands, cupping her breasts, and fondling her clitoris.

HIS O-METER ★★★☆☆

With this sex position, there's not much in the way for him to look at, which can be a bummer during sex. Fix this by installing a mirror next to your bed if you don't already have one. He can enter her from behind, while still getting to enjoy checking her out from top to bottom.

MAKE IT HOTTER . . .

This is the perfect position for spontaneous middle-of-the-night sex. To add a BDSM twist, he can pull her hair, or grab her throat from behind.

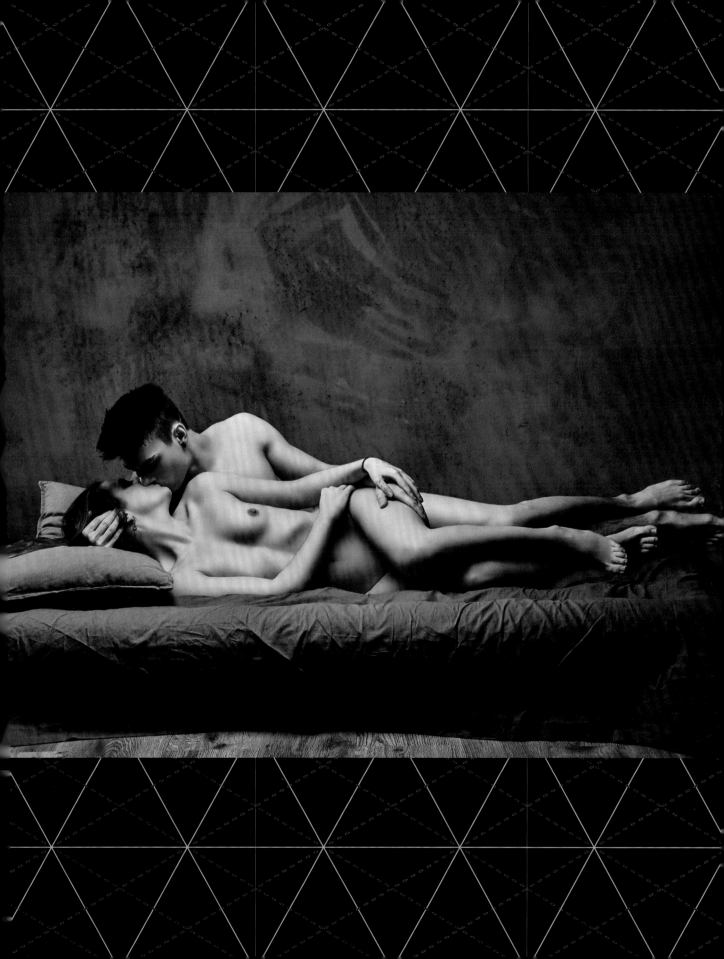

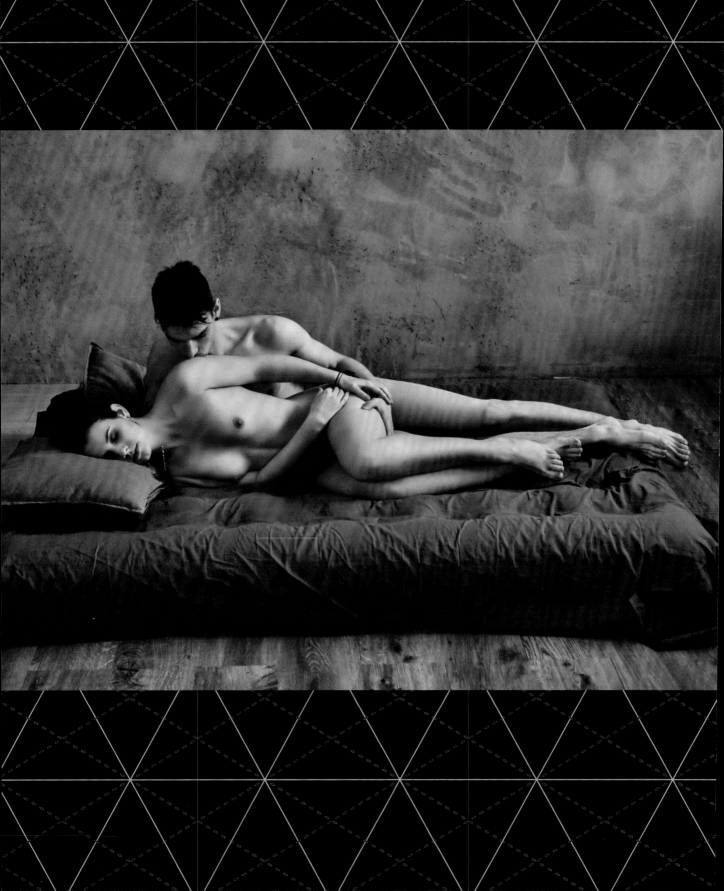

SPORK

The Spork is a sweetly intimate, side-by-side sex position you can use for rear-entry vaginal sex or even anal sex if you like. A must try!

HOW TO DO IT

Assume the traditional spooning sex position (see page 192), with both partners lying on their sides, and the male partner resting the front of his torso and groin against his partner's back and rear end. Instead of leaving her legs straight, as in the spooning sex position, the female partner will draw her legs all the way up against her chest so she is in the fetal position. Her partner will draw his legs up slightly to curve around her body, and will wrap his arms around her torso.

WHERE TO DO IT

The bed is, of course, the easiest place to do the Spork, but feel free to get creative. Try it on a picnic blanket out in the middle of a field, or in the back of a pickup truck!

PROPS YOU'LL NEED

None.

DIFFICULTY LEVEL ★☆☆☆☆

HER O-METER ★☆☆☆☆

The Spork isn't as exciting for her as other sex positions because her clitoris is almost completely non-accessible, and her G-spot doesn't get much action either. This is more of a novelty for her than anything else.

HIS O-METER ★★★☆☆

He enjoys the intimacy of the Spork, as well as the rear entry angle. However, he doesn't get much of a view here and can't really see what is going on, so his visual system isn't going to be as stimulated as it is with other sex positions where he can watch the action.

MAKE IT HOTTER...

She can turn her head to gaze deeply into his eyes and make a soulful, intimate connection during lovemaking. He can also reach around and fondle her breasts and nipples.

TWISTER

If you're looking for a super-exotic sex position, the Twister should be right up your alley. Challenging, yet fun—it's a must try!

HOW TO DO IT

The female partner lies on her right side, and her partner also lies on his right side, facing away from her. He will be positioned with his head to her feet and his feet to her head. Both partners will bend their left knees and lift them up, to create a space where their groins can come together to facilitate penetration. This ends up with both partners in between each other's legs. Sound complicated? It can be, but if you check out the picture on the next page, it may be a little easier to figure it out.

WHERE TO DO IT

The bed is the best place for the Twister sex position, since it requires space and is so complicated to get into. You definitely don't want to be worrying about logistics when you're busy figuring out how to thrust!

PROPS YOU'LL NEED

Both partners may appreciate some pillows, but they're not necessary.

DIFFICULTY LEVEL ★★★★★

HER O-METER ★★★★☆

The Twister sex position allows her to grind her clitoris against him during penetration, increasing her orgasm potential and overall satisfaction. This may not be her favorite sex position, but it's easier for her to orgasm in this one than in many other "exotic" sex positions.

HIS O-METER ★★★★☆

The angle of penetration and the ability for him to thrust in the Twister sex position is a bit difficult for him, but he definitely likes the novelty of this one. He'll want to try it for sure, but it may not end up being his favorite either.

MAKE IT HOTTER . . .

Focus on getting a rhythm down with the Twister sex position, and getting more experienced at it, instead of worrying about how to make it hotter. If you can accomplish this sex position and stay in it for any length of time, you're doing well!

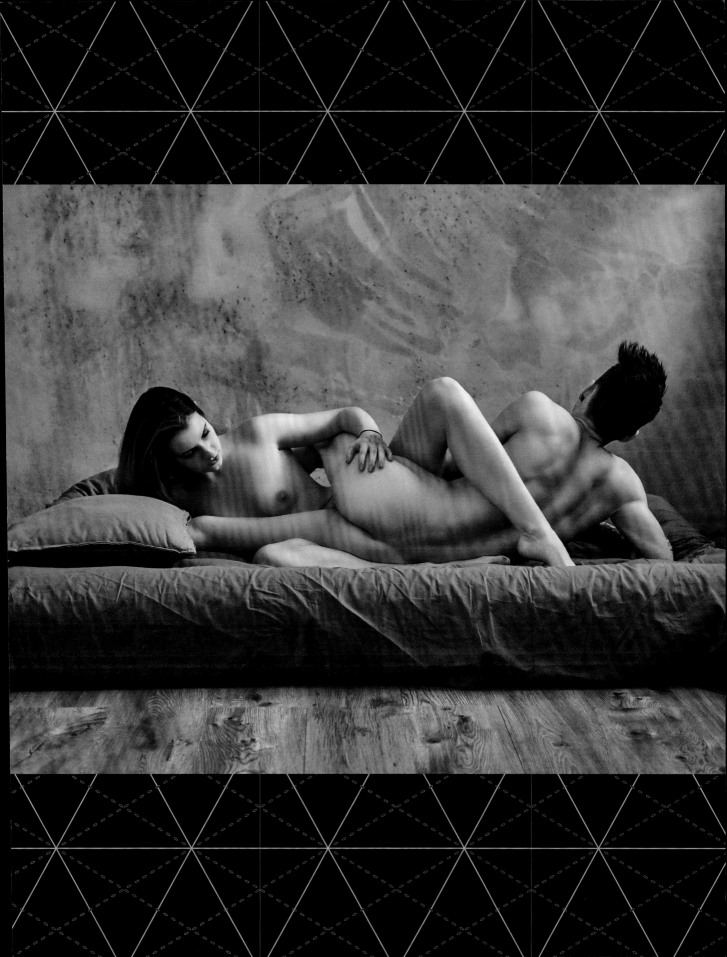

SEXY CHALLENGE:

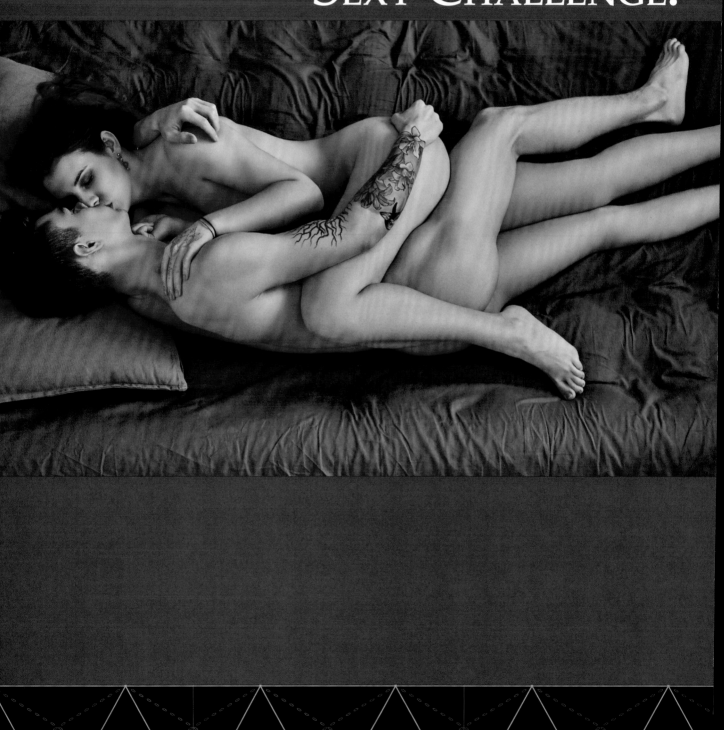

THE EQUALS SIGN

Most sexual positions have a dominant partner and a submissive partner, if you will; one partner is in control of the thrusting and movements, while the other partner is limited in the movements and engagements they can make. This Sexy Challenge, called The Equal sign, is designed around the side-by-side positions in this chapter of the book. The challenge really focuses on the beauty of a couple working together to bring pleasure to both partners through orgasm, allowing for more touching, more connection, and more stimulation together.

Think of the equal sign: it is two straight lines running side by side, and in mathematical terms it means that both numbers or equations on the opposite sides of the equal sign represent the same value. While the man-on-top positions are focused on pleasure for the man mostly, and the woman-on top positions are focused on the woman mostly, we want to give you a chance to experience the same amount or equal pleasure together. Now, while there are various positions listed in the side-by-side position section, we want to focus on the ones that allow you to have face-to-face contact with your partner, such as the Crazy Starfish position.

While the goal of sex is usually to bring each other to orgasm and/or climax, we want a little different approach here. Yes, don't worry, you are going to get off. These positions provide a window for play that is unique. So, we are going to take you on a ride that will end in an amazing orgasm, but along the way, you are going to be treated to some sensations that most people bypass on their way to that blissful orgasm. You have heard the phrase, "Stop and smell the roses." Well, we are going to allow you to smell, touch, lick, kiss, fondle, and squeeze the roses all the way to the climactic end.

The first thing you need to do is set aside plenty of time for this Sexy Challenge. Stopping and smelling the roses is about experiencing all you can, and if you are going to be rushed, that is not going to happen. Next, prepare in advance for all the things you might need while in the equal sign of sex positions. Once you get started, you are not going to want to get up to get lubrication, prophylactics, or anything else that might throw you off balance, or out of the equal sign mentality. Next, you need to get your mind in the right place, and together you can meditate on this, or just understand that you are both equal partners in bringing the pleasure. So, that means you stimulate yourself as well as your partner, and vice versa. The one stipulation in this Sexy Challenge is that you stimulate yourself as well as your partner.

Time to get into the Crazy Starfish Position. As you join together, take a moment to bask in the beauty of your partner. While you are connected, look and enjoy his/her beauty. Stare deep into each other's eyes and feel the equal sign that you have become. Think about this at this moment in time when you are connected as one: you are equal because you are just one living being at this time. You have joined together and are now a blended spirit. You are sharing space, sharing heartbeats, and sharing the portal to divine pleasure. If that doesn't get you turned on, I am not sure what will. Bask in this glory for just a moment or two, continue to stare into your partner's eyes, and now send them messages with your mind about the pleasure you would like to receive. Put your sexy visions into their mind, and allow them to put their sexy vision into your mind. You might have a mental orgasm at this point, and that is okay; mind orgasms will help going forward. Even a man can rejuvenate from a mind orgasm easily.

Now, let's start adding more power to this equally turned on, connected being that is our equal sign. Like boiling water, stimulation will start to make things hotter and hotter in your equals-sign encounter. Stimulating yourself in the throes of passion might be a little more difficult for the men, as most women that are very sexual do this already. So, I am going to share some things you need to incorporate into the play, and all of them you can do to yourself or your partner. Remember, you are equals now, and whatever you do to pleasure yourself will benefit not only you, but your partner, too. In the following paragraphs are a list of areas to consider for play. Again, you can play with your own body or your partner's. Allow the flow of the equal sign to direct your hands, mouth, tongue, etc., where they need to go. Remember, we can't possibly touch on all areas, but let's cover the basics.

In the Crazy Starfish position, you have access to your body and your partner's, so reach out and touch yourself and your partner in some of these areas. To begin with, know that the skin is your largest erogenous zone, and that touching any part of the body can light up sensors in the brain that will quickly be relayed to the genitals. Nipples can be the volume controls for pleasure, so reach out and see if you or your partner's nipples are erect. If not, see if you can change that. Now, while this position is a little difficult for much kissing, that doesn't mean you can't stick your fingers in your partner's mouth, or kiss and lick those fingers. Don't forget you both have an anus and they are very sensitive to touch with all those nerve endings, so feel free to rub your own anus or your partner's in this position. This position also allows you both access to the clitoris on the ladies and the scrotum on the men. Share the touching with your partner in both these areas, and watch things start to really heat up.

The Equals-Sign Sexy Challenge is all about sharing and caring: sharing your pleasure, and caring that your partner has equal amounts of pleasure. As you go through this process and experience the orgasms and climaxes that come with it, take the time to keep looking into the eyes of your partner and see the pleasure you are enjoying reflected in their eyes. Soak in the experience of watching the pleasure your partner is receiving, and allow them to watch the pleasure wash over you. After you experience this equal lovemaking, you will be forever changed. Each kiss, each touch, and each encounter going forward will be an exciting sharing of equal pleasure.

Other things you can consider bringing into this Equals-Sign Sexy Challenge would be toys, especially vibrators. Yes, men can get turned on from the feel of a vibrator, as well as the women. Anal plugs and beads can be equally exciting for both men and women during this experience. Some couples might even like to bring food into the fun, while others might like to play with a flogger, or enjoy some spanking while being equal. Heck, you might even enjoy a glass of wine during the festivities, or a shot of whiskey; the choice is yours together. The goal is to bring an equal amount of pleasure to the both of you. For when the pleasure is shared equally, the pleasure moves from great to amazing, or even to OMFG!

CHAPTER 9 : DEEP-PENETRATION SEX POSITIONS

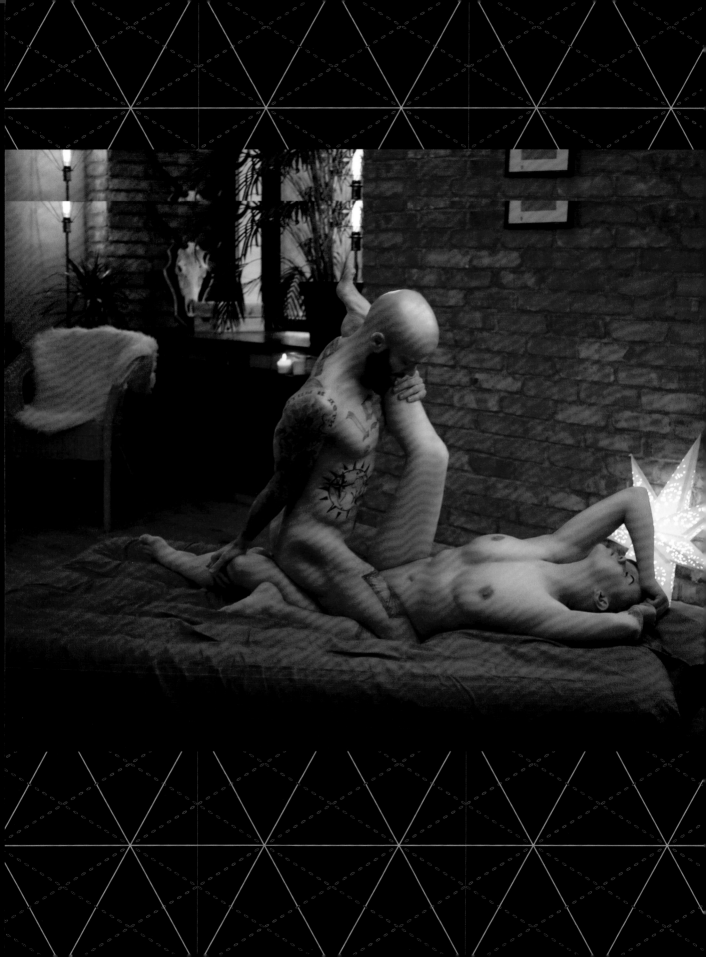

CLIMBING THE FLAGPOLE

The Climbing-the-Flagpole sex position is a deep-penetration twist on Missionary that is great for both partners. It's comfortable for most women, yet totally erotic and orgasmic! There's not too much strain on either partner, as long as she is fairly flexible, and the view for both is incredible.

HOW TO DO IT

The female partner lies on her side, as though she's about to be spooned, and supports her head with her hand. The male partner straddles her leg that is resting on the bed and lifts the other, so that it rests against his chest and her foot is pointed straight up towards the ceiling. To make this a bit more comfortable for her, she can add a slight bend to her knee without compromising this position at all. He will do the majority of the thrusting here.

WHERE TO DO IT

This is another sex position that requires some space if both partners are to be as comfortable as possible, so the bed or floor are good choices.

PROPS YOU'LL NEED

She will definitely want a pillow under her head if you are going to keep up the Climbing-the-Flagpole sex position for any length of time.

DIFFICULTY LEVEL ★★☆☆☆

HER O-METER ★★★☆☆

He can grind against her clitoris fairly well in this position, making it much better for her. The deeper penetration is also good for G-spot or even A-spot orgasms!

HIS O-METER ★★★★☆

He really enjoys the view in this position. He likes that she's spread wide open for him, and that he can look down and see everything that is going on. A bit more exotic than the average sex position, Climbing the Flagpole looks more difficult than it actually is. He can thrust fairly well without too much strain on his body.

MAKE IT HOTTER . . .

This is a great sex position for either him or her to reach down and play with her clitoris! This makes the Climbing the Flagpole much more satisfying for her.

CRADLE

The Cradle is definitely considered an "exotic" sex position, and it can be a little difficult to master, but is highly rewarding if you do. The female partner needs to be fairly flexible, but if she can bend in this position, it gives her partner a great show and the perfect angle for nipple or clitoral play.

HOW TO DO IT

The male partner kneels and rests his rear on his feet. The female partner straddles his pelvis and then bends backwards with the help of her lover's hands supporting her lower back. When the position has been achieved, it will look almost exactly like the Bridge (see page 322) with the female partner's hands resting on the floor and her back arched, but with her buttocks resting on her partner's legs instead. This sex position is a little easier for the female partner, yet lends an "exotic feel."

WHERE TO DO IT

The floor is ideal for this position, but a firm bed will work as well.

PROPS YOU'LL NEED

A soft blanket or thick towel to go under his knees for comfort.

DIFFICULTY LEVEL ★★★★☆

HER O-METER ★☆☆☆☆

While this sex position is a little more comfortable than the Bridge, it only allows for slightly more clitoral friction. This makes it a little easier for her to reach orgasm, but not much. With lots of foreplay beforehand, however, her partner can make sure she's turned on enough to have a better chance of reaching the big O.

HIS O-METER ★★★☆☆

While supporting her weight on his thighs might be a little awkward for him, the main issue here is for a man with a smaller penis. Since his thighs are pressed together, only a bigger penis will have enough length to penetrate his partner fully. If this position can be achieved well, however, he will enjoy the view. It might be a little difficult for him to thrust, though.

MAKE IT HOTTER . . .

Guys, spread your legs a little wider to allow your penis more room to penetrate. You might have to support your girl's hips a little more if your legs are spread, but it will be well worth it!

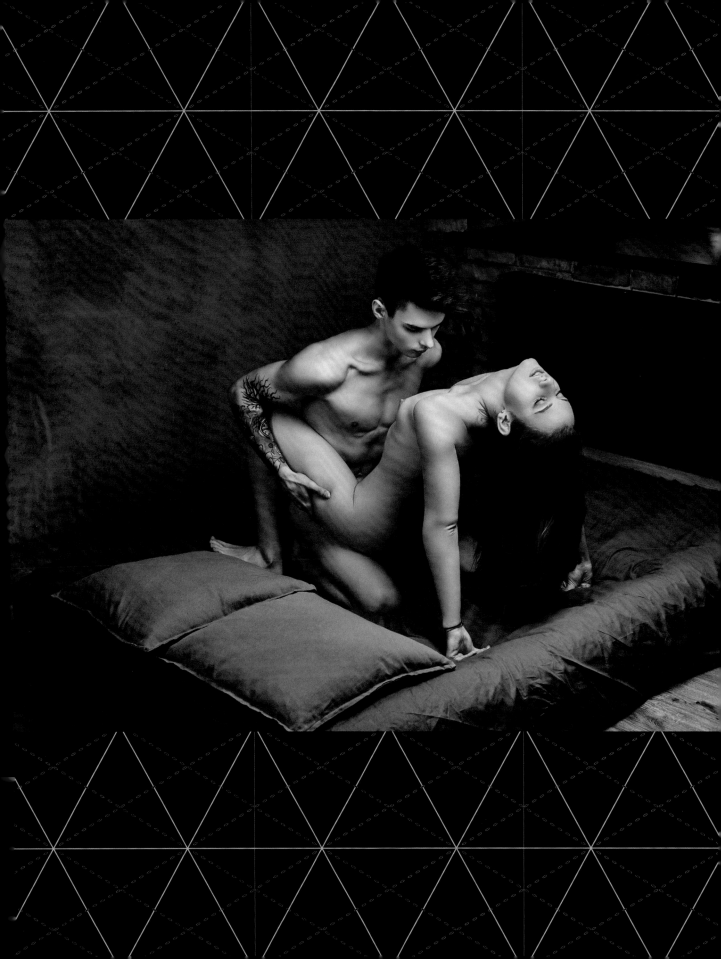

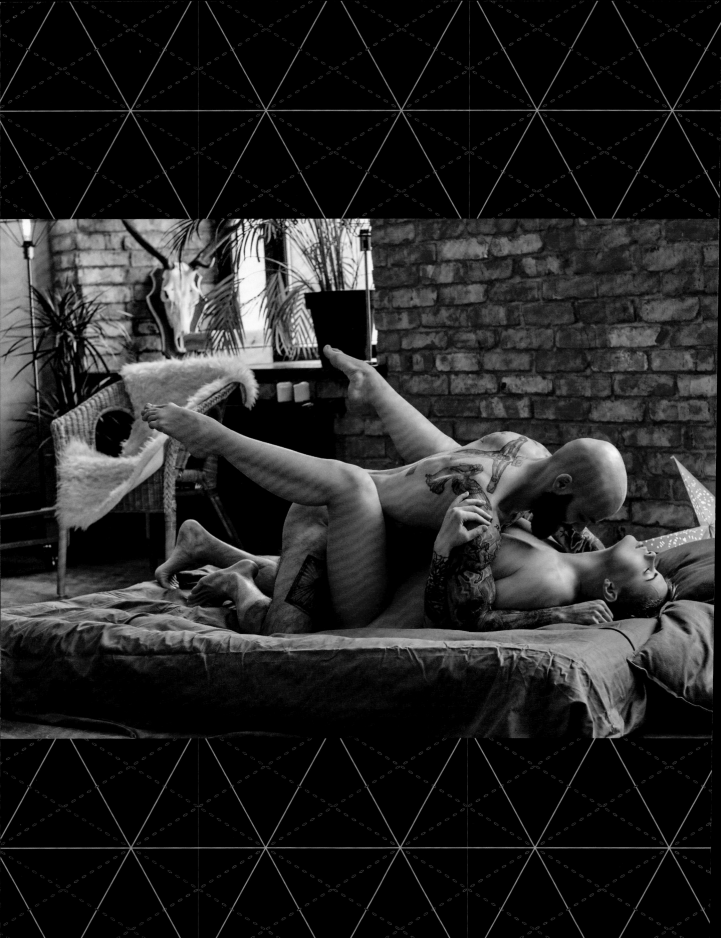

DECK CHAIR

The Deck Chair sex position is a deep penetration twist on Missionary that both partners will really enjoy! It's simple to do, but deeply satisfying for both partners. Get the deep sensations of Doggy Style (see page 244) or Rear Entry (see page 240) with the eye contact and intimacy of the Missionary sex position.

HOW TO DO IT

The Deck Chair is very similar to the Missionary, except for where the female partner places her legs. In this position, she raises her thighs to a ninety-degree angle, without hooking them around his backside or resting them on his shoulders. This position is really great for G-spot or even A-spot stimulation because it facilitates much deeper penetration than the Missionary position does.

WHERE TO DO IT

The Deck Chair can be done just about anywhere that you have room to lie down.

PROPS YOU'LL NEED

A pillow for her lower back can make this position more comfortable, especially if you do it on the floor. It will also help tilt the pelvis for even deeper G-spot and A-spot penetration.

DIFFICULTY LEVEL ★☆☆☆☆

HER O-METER ★★★★☆

She loves this sex position because it gives her a much better angle for G-spot stimulation. It's much more likely that her partner will rub her just the right way in the Deck Chair position than in the traditional Missionary. She can spread her legs a little or a lot depending on her mood.

HIS O-METER ★★★★☆

If she gets off, he gets off. Enough said.

MAKE IT HOTTER...

Take it up a notch and bring her feet up as high possible for some super deep penetration. It's OK for her to bend her knees. Make sure to take it slow because not all women love contact to the cervix.

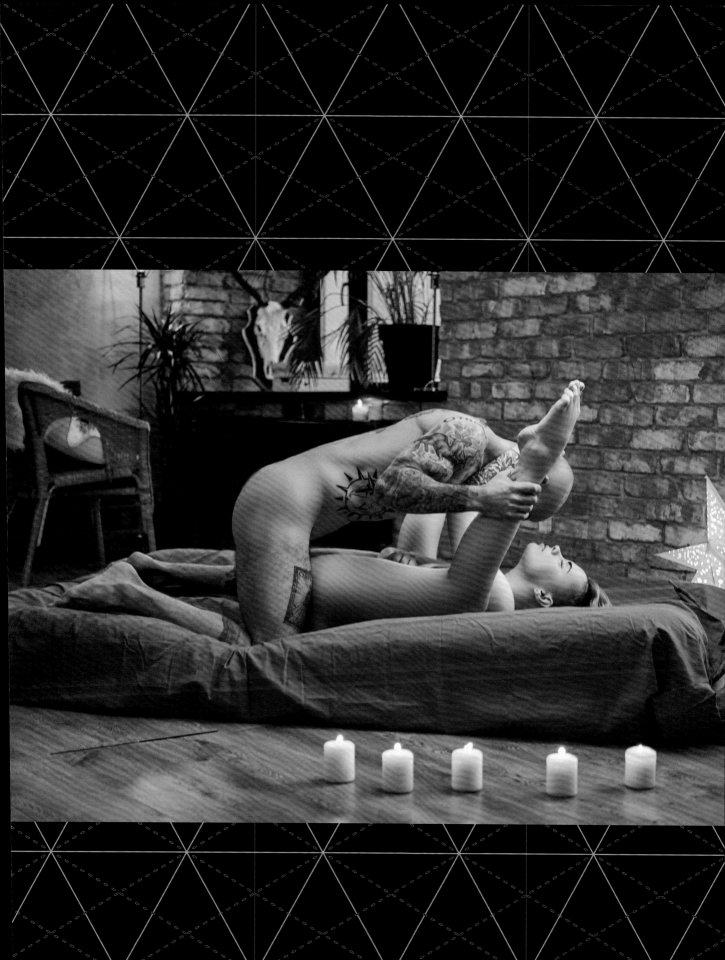

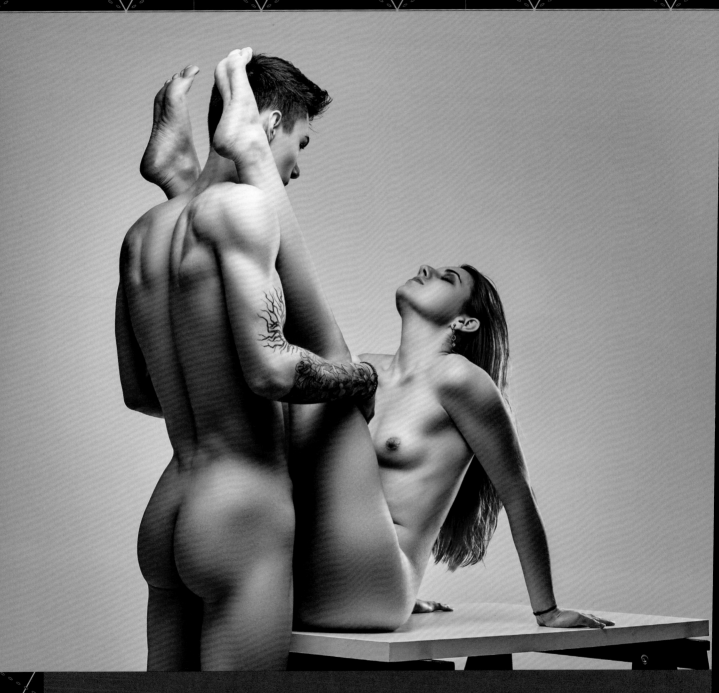

MAKE IT HOTTER . . .

Save the Deep-Victory sex position for laundry day and do it on top of the washer during the spin cycle. The vibrations will drive you both absolutely insane! Talk about hot!

DEEP VICTORY

The Deep-Victory sex position is a bit difficult for women who aren't flexible, but if you can do this one, the deep penetration and intimacy are worth it! It's an excellent sex position for G-spot and A-spot stimulation, and the face-to-face contact makes this one a must try.

HOW TO DO IT

The female partner sits on a surface like a countertop or table that is roughly level with her partner's groin. He will stand and pull her legs up over his shoulders before entering her, and her feet and ankles will be resting on either side of his neck. Again, this can be a very difficult position to get into because it's more suited to athletic women who are quite flexible.

WHERE TO DO IT

Any surface that is level with the male partner's groin will work for this position.

PROPS YOU'LL NEED

If he is on the short side, or the surface you're using is on the high side, he may need a footstool to get himself high up enough to facilitate comfortable penetration. She may also want a towel, soft blanket, or pillow under her rear.

DIFFICULTY LEVEL ★★★★☆

HER O-METER ★☆☆☆☆

If she's not flexible, she's not going to like the Deep-Victory sex position very much at all. It will be awkward and uncomfortable for her, and she may not be able to continue in the position for very long. However, if she's an athletic girl with flexible legs, this sex position really isn't going to be that difficult for her. If you can get into this position comfortably, don't skip out on it, because the G-spot stimulation in the Deep-Victory sex position is incredible!

HIS O-METER ★★★★☆

He loves this sex position because it's easy for him to get into, and it's on the exotic side, without being over the top. He can't really watch what is going on down there, but he loves the way she is spread out and waiting for him. He digs the deep penetration too, and he won't be able to last long in this position!

G-FORCE

In the G-Force sex position, deep penetration is achieved in a unique way. It can be uncomfortable for the woman, but it's also really hot!

HOW TO DO IT

The male partner kneels in front of the female partner, who is on her back, with her knees together and drawn up towards her chest. He then lifts her hips up to meet his and enters her, with her feet either flat on his chest or in his hands. This interesting sex position can be used for either vaginal intercourse or anal sex, although it's not a good position for anal sex beginners. If you're just starting out with anal play, try another sex position first.

WHERE TO DO IT

G-Force can be done on the bed, sofa, floor, or even the car if you've got a big enough back seat! Just remember that the G-Force can be rough on a woman's neck and upper back, so make sure you keep her comfort in mind.

PROPS YOU'LL NEED

She will really appreciate a pillow under her head and possibly one under her shoulders. If you're doing this position on the floor, lay down a blanket or towel first. Carpet burns hurt!

DIFFICULTY LEVEL ★★★★☆

HER O-METER ★★★☆☆

It can be a bit uncomfortable with the awkward angle created in the neck and shoulders area, but with proper support like a pillow or rolled-up towel, she should be able to stay in this sex position for a decent amount of time. It definitely allows for super-deep penetration, which many women will enjoy!

HIS O-METER ★★★★★

He absolutely loves the G-Force sex position, because he gets to see pretty much everything! It's just as good as the Reverse Cowgirl (see page 57) in terms of how much he enjoys the show. The deep penetration is nice for him too, and if he gets to do anal like this, he'll be totally stoked.

MAKE IT HOTTER . . .

He can hold her feet in his hands to control the angle of penetration and the spread of her legs.

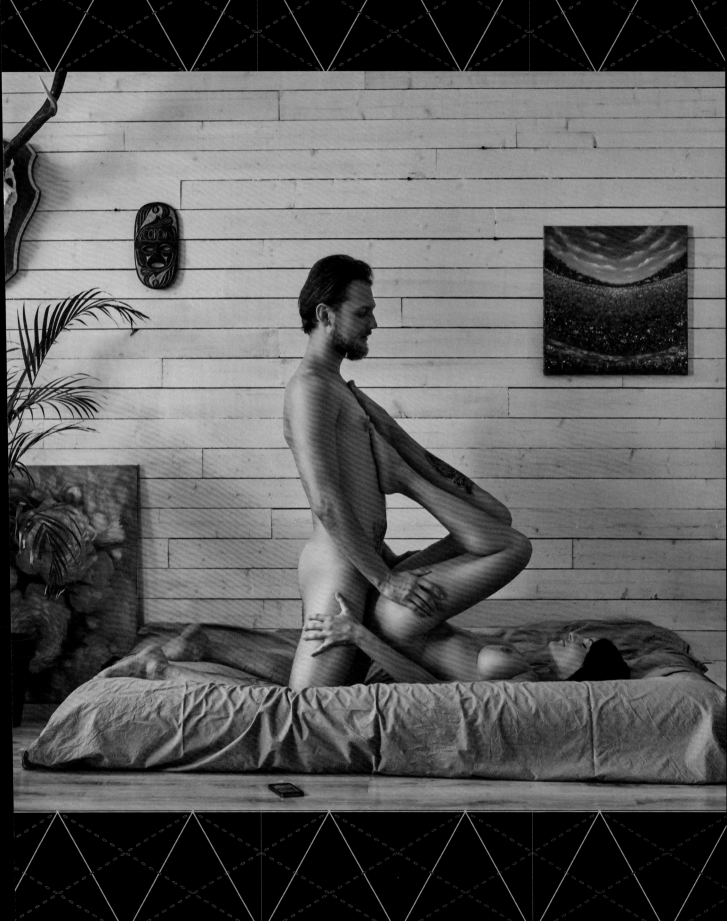

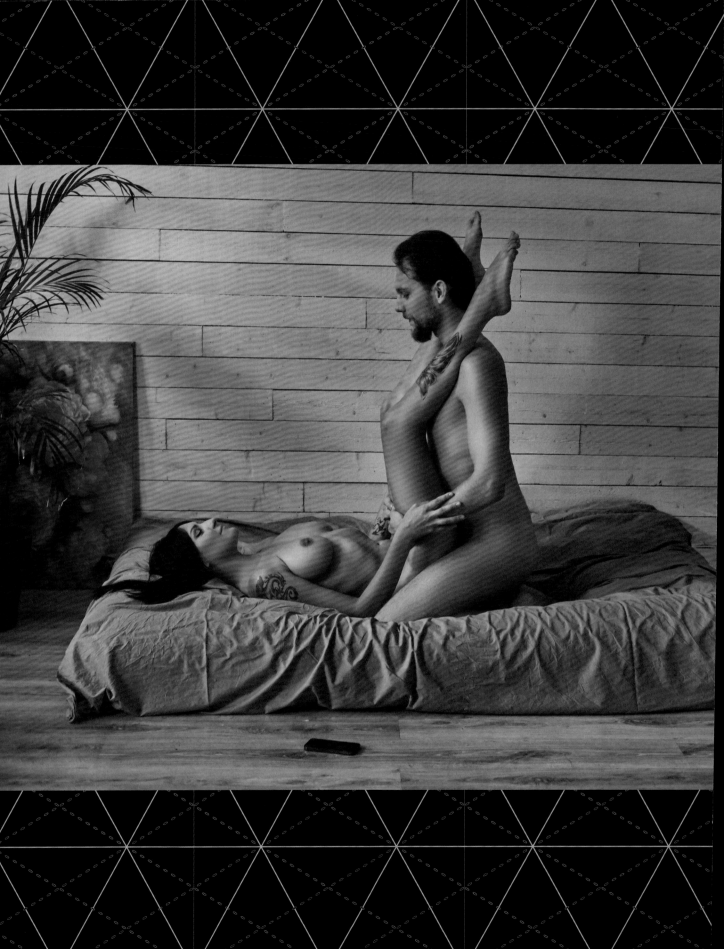

SHOULDER HOLDER

Get the deepest possible penetration and awesome G-spot stimulation with the Shoulder Holder sex position! You really can't get any deeper than this, and the stimulation feels great for both partners.

HOW TO DO IT

The Shoulder Holder is another twist on the Missionary, but is a little more challenging. The female partner rests on her back with her legs straight up in the air, and the male partner sits up on his knees to penetrate her. Her legs will rest gently on his shoulders. This move can be a little more difficult for women who aren't as flexible in the legs. Ladies, feel free to bend your knees gently, if your legs begin to feel too stretched.

WHERE TO DO IT

The Shoulder Holder can be done pretty much anywhere that you can do the Missionary. Try the bed, floor, sofa, and even the recliner!

PROPS YOU'LL NEED

None.

DIFFICULTY LEVEL ★★★☆☆

HER O-METER ★★★★☆

The Shoulder Holder allows for the deepest penetration. She can fully feel him inside of her, and he can reach her A-spot easily in this position. With plenty of foreplay and clitoral stimulation, she can achieve a really intense orgasm in this position.

HIS O-METER ★★★★☆

He will love the view in this sex position! It's another sex position in which he is the dominant partner, and this can be exceptionally erotic for him. He can grab her legs or hips and use them as leverage to thrust even deeper. He will really enjoy being able to feel every inch of himself inside her.

MAKE IT HOTTER . . .

To give him a super sexy view, she can spread her legs in a "V." This allows him to see and enjoy all the hot, sweaty action!

VIENNESE OYSTER

The Viennese-Oyster sex position is deliciously naughty, although it is difficult to master for most women. However, if you can, the rewards are great!

HOW TO DO IT

The female partner lies on her back, raises her legs, and wraps them behind her head and crosses her ankles. Of course, this is quite a difficult position for women who aren't extremely flexible! It allows her partner to enter her quite easily because her entire groin is exposed. He should be resting his weight on his hands, instead of on his partner. He can even distribute some of his weight onto his knees to make it easier on both partners.

If the female partner has trouble getting her feet to rest all the way behind her head, this position can also be achieved fairly well by simply having her partner push her legs down enough so that each ankle is on either side of her head. (This would be a modified version of the Viennese-Oyster sex position).

WHERE TO DO IT

She needs lots of space for this one so a nice, big bed is the best choice.

PROPS YOU'LL NEED

None.

DIFFICULTY LEVEL ★★★★★

HER O-METER ★☆☆☆☆

The Viennese-Oyster sex position is going to be more difficult for her than pleasurable, unless she's very flexible. If she is not flexible, this position will be fairly awkward for her, and she's not going to be able to keep it up for an extended period of time. For her, this sex position is more of a novelty than anything else. For those select few women who are quite flexible, the star-rating on this one goes way up! He can penetrate her deeply and the angle increases G-spot stimulation for some very intense orgasms.

HIS O-METER ★★★★★

It's unfortunate for him that she doesn't really get off in the Viennese-Oyster sex position, because he loves it. She is completely and totally spread out for his pleasure, and the feeling of his penis sliding in and out of her without her thighs, or anything else getting in the way, can't be beat.

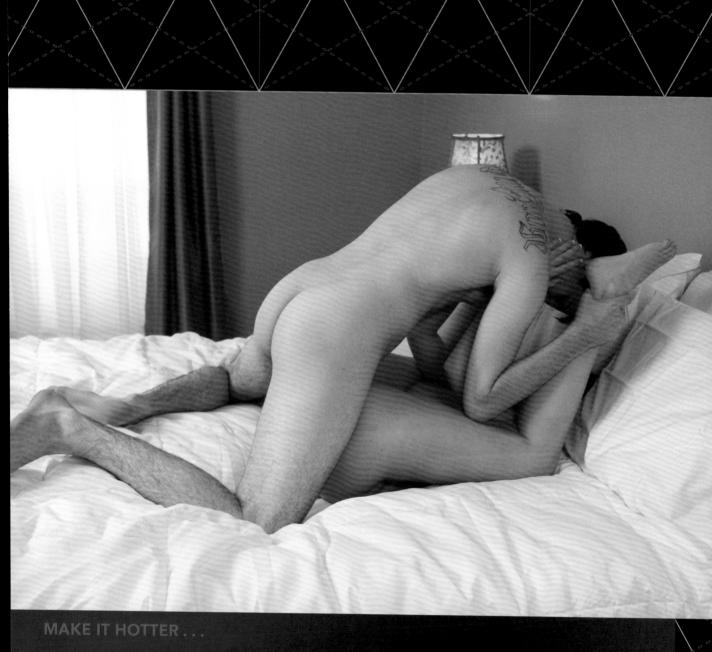

MAKE IT HOTTER . . .

This sex position is super-hot already, and there's not much else you can do when you're occupied like this.

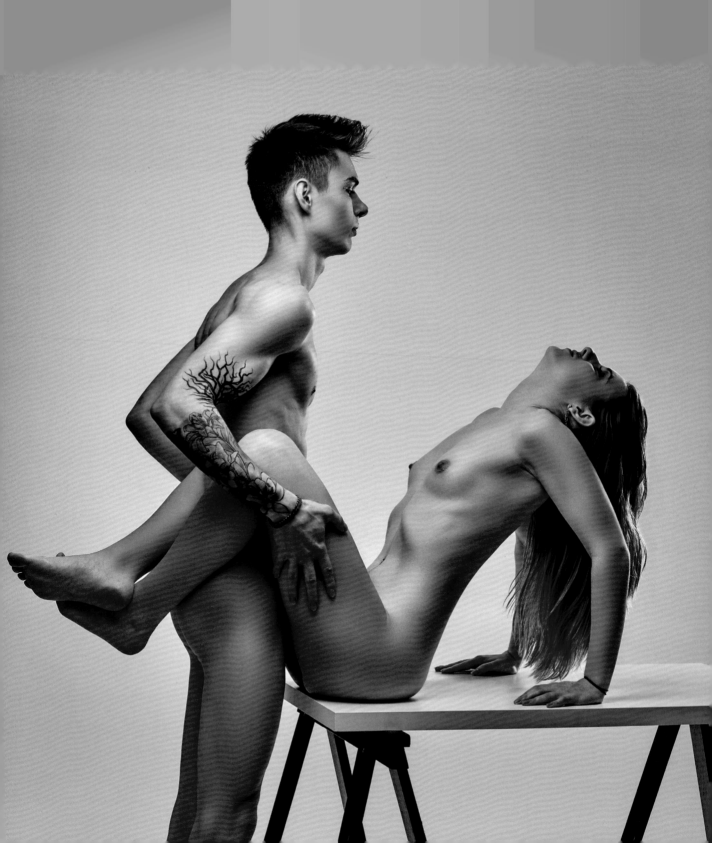

Sex can take you many places, and I am not talking about amazing vacations. I am talking about places where you can witness things that you can't otherwise: spiritual places, metaphysical places, past-life experiences, and even distant planets, to name a few. Sex is a gateway to the cosmos. The pleasure is a doorway to dimensions that we cannot explain, but we love going to. Think about that moment of orgasm or climax and how your mind is so engorged in pleasure that it checks out for that brief, but pleasurable, moment. Where does your mind or your consciousness go? While we cannot explain it, and it might even be different for each and every one of us, we do know that it is a magical place. I consider this brief moment in our time as a Star Voyage: a fast blast out to the ends of the cosmos and back again. That is why we are tired and worn out when we come back. Sure, some might say it is the sex that wears us out, but if you really think about it . . . you will know it is much, much more than that.

The problem is that we as humans don't allow our mind to experience all the pleasures of the sexual experience. We are so focused on our partner and our pleasure that we forget to pay attention. Why the fuck do humans do this? We are so focused on the goal that we miss the real enjoyment that happens all around us on the path. Well, this Star-Voyage Sexy Challenge is going to help you witness the beauty, the ideas, the energy, and the total experience of what sex is supposed to be. This is the perfect Sexy Challenge to couple with the Deep-Penetration Positions that have just been shared with you. I hate to use this statement, but by opening your mind during these deep penetrative sexual positions, you will be able to "Boldly Go Where No Man or Woman has Gone Before." Sorry, but you could have gone there before; you just didn't pay attention. So, set your phasers on stun, and prepare for takeoff.

The Deep-Penetration sex position allows you to touch parts of your partner that don't get touched very often. Most normal sex positions are designed to stimulate different pleasure zones, and unless the man is extremely well-endowed, it's not going to touch those deep sections. The deep penetrative positions allow us to experience different sensations and pleasures, so they are perfect for our Star-Voyage Sexy Challenge. During sex there are many, many things happening around you that you are most likely not aware of, like the release of new and amazing energy. Yes, I know we have all heard that energy cannot be created or destroyed, but that is crap. Sex creates energy, sex creates life, sex creates so many things it is crazy. Being open enough to experience these things is the trick.

It has been one of the greatest pleasures in my life to be able to witness and view the sexual energy I have helped to create. It is like witnessing the creation of a work of art. When you create sexual energy, you are giving yourself a creative license to be a more incredible version of yourself. So, in our Star Voyage, you will learn the tips and tricks for witnessing the energy you have helped to create. I personally believe that if we create enough powerful sexual energy, we can change major things in our universe. It can stop wars, feed the hungry, heal our planet, and the list goes on and on. But the first step is to get you to where you can see the sexual energy and the visions that come along with it. Yes, there are visions that come along with this sexual energy, visions that actually help you create a better life for yourself. This has all been happening for you, and you have been missing it.

As humans, we are focused on the task at hand, so when we are having sex, sex is our focus. Our minds are on one track, and that track is usually getting to orgasm, which is a lovely place. However, our minds are amazing and can focus on more than one thing at a time. So, as you begin your journey with your lover and get into a deep penetrative sexual position like the Bridge, I want you to take some deep meditative breaths. Allow air to flow into your lungs, and out your genitals, and into your partner. This opens the passage for the messages to become clear. Breathing during this entire process is important, so even as you climax and orgasm, try to keep the breathing up. Most of us tend to quit breathing at the moment of orgasm, as we are trying to hold on to the feeling, but try to breathe through it. As you breathe, images will start to pop into your mind, as the air and the sexual energy begin to combine. Now, we don't want you to stop and take notes as you are having sex, but we do want you to be aware of things that stick out to you during this process. Make a mental note of anything you witness in your mind while this is happening. It is OK to blurt words out during this sexual experience; tell your lover to do the same.

As you near climax, focus on your breathing and don't try to hold back the flow of orgasmic pleasure; let it flow with your breathing. Be very aware at this point, for this is when the big messages will come through. They will be cryptic, in the sense that you have to figure out what they mean. However, with a little thought, you will be able to figure out what they mean to you. Now, you might physically see things, or you might just have a sense of them; either way, that is powerful. After all is said and done with your sexual experience, you both need to take the time to jot down your experience to review later. I even suggest keeping a Star-Voyage Journal by the bed, because you might start to see connections each time you do this Star Voyage. I will also say that each time you do this process, it gets easier and easier and you get more information. That doesn't mean every session is amazing; just like sex, sometimes it isn't as good as the last time, but it doesn't stop you from trying it again.

There are some things you can do to help the process of your Star-Voyage Sexy Challenge. First of all, many people find alcohol helps relax them to have this experience and while that is OK, too much alcohol can also dampen the experience. The same goes for any drugs; since marijuana is legal in some places now, it might be something you could use to relax yourself enough to witness this experience. Apple juice is another great way to help experience the Star Voyage, just as it helps in bringing on dreams—for some, it may act as a lubricant for your visions to come through. Meditation and/or a massage beforehand can also be a big help to get you in the mood to receive these messages from the cosmos. You can experiment around also to see what might work for you; some people use music to help, others take a relaxing bath beforehand, and others might do yoga. The beauty is, there is no exact answer, so you can always be looking for something new and fun to try out in the process.

I do feel it is important for you to keep a journal and write down all your experiences. Even if you don't have any experiences, write down what you did before the deep penetrative position you tried, and any other outside factors that could be an issue. Once you get in the habit of keeping good notes on your Star Voyages, you can start looking back and seeing if there might be connections between experiences. By doing this, sometimes those cryptic messages start to become more and more clear. The most beautiful part of this is that you get to have amazing and creative deep penetrative sex, create amazing sexual energy with your lover, and possibly get the secrets that will make your life as amazing as possible. You might even get messages that will help humankind boldly go where no one has gone before.

CHAPTER 10: 69 SEX POSITIONS

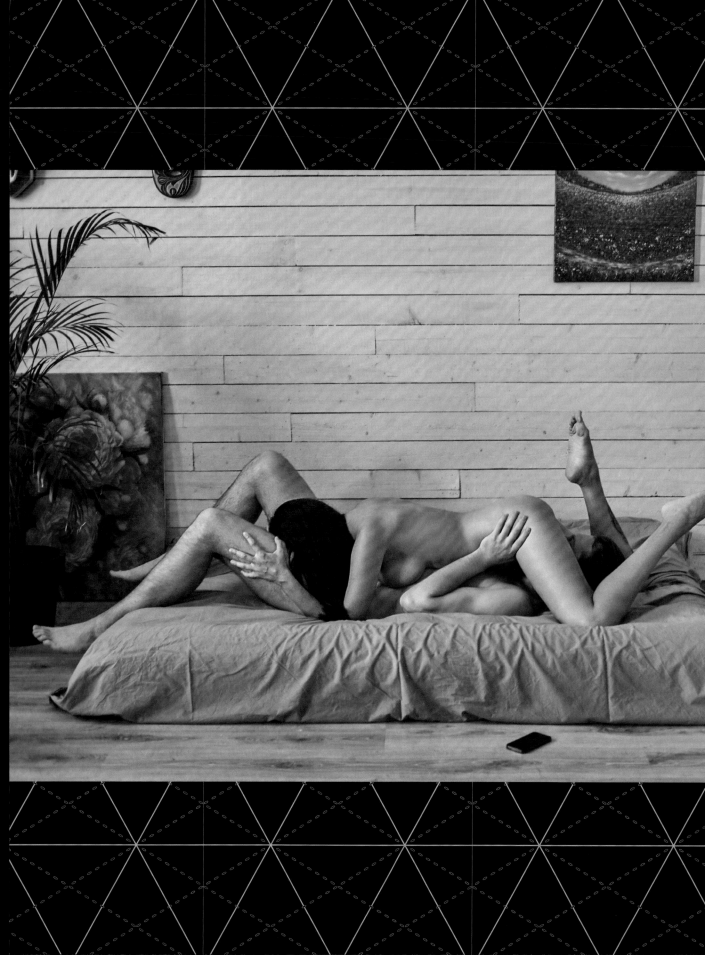

Traditionally, the 69 is one of the most exciting ways to give and receive oral sex, because both partners get do it at the same time. This is a great way to bring each other to simultaneous orgasm orally, and it can be a great position to use when one partner is less enthusiastic about giving oral sex.

HOW TO DO IT

In the 69, the male partner lies on a flat surface on his back, and the female partner straddles his face, facing towards his feet. She then leans down and performs oral sex on him, while simultaneously receiving it.

For the 69 to be successful, however, both partners must be clean and very comfortable with each other. The partner on top may feel exposed, since her lover's mouth and nose are so close to her buttocks and genitals. Don't forget to do some basic hygiene beforehand (such as a sexy shower together), and you shouldn't have any issues.

WHERE TO DO IT

You can do the 69 on the floor, sofa, bed, reclining chair, outdoors, or anywhere you can both comfortably lie down.

PROPS YOU'LL NEED

None.

DIFFICULTY LEVEL ★☆☆☆☆

HER O-METER ★★★★☆

The 69 is a great way for a woman to receive oral sex when her partner is reluctant to go down on her without getting anything in return. By offering to do the 69, she can entice her lover to do something for her, because she's doing something for him. Some guys enjoy performing oral sex on a woman regardless, but other men have difficulty enjoying oral sex if they're not being stimulated in some way as well. The only caveat here is that she's focusing on giving him oral pleasure, so her own is reduced somewhat. She cannot fully focus on the sensations and pleasure of receiving oral sex, simply because she's trying to do two things at once.

HIS O-METER ★★★★☆

Guys like the idea of being able to receive oral sex at the same time they give it, because for some men, giving oral sex isn't enjoyable in and of itself, if they're not being stimulated in some way. The 69 is an excellent solution to this problem! However, he cannot focus solely on his own pleasure, because he's also trying to give her oral pleasure as well. It's definitely enjoyable for him, but just slightly less enjoyable than if he were to be able to sit back, relax, and enjoy a blowjob.

MAKE IT HOTTER...

Take your time and enjoy giving each other oral sex. Learning to move in sync and communicate sexually without speaking to each other can be extremely sexy and intimate!

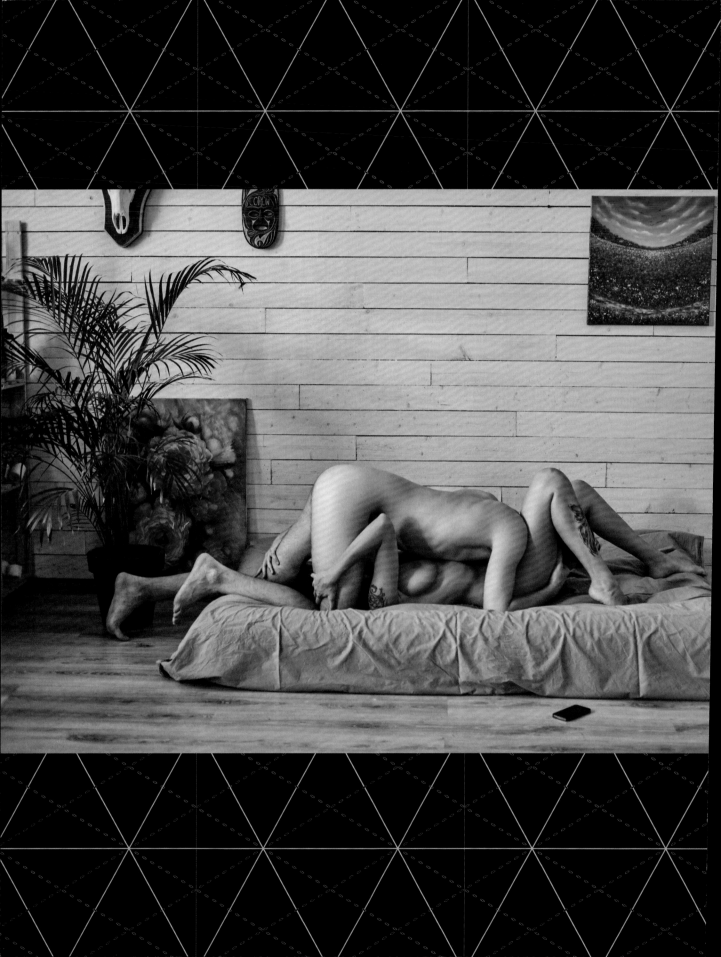

REVERSE 69

If the 69 sex position is one of the most exciting ways to give and receive oral sex, the Reverse-69 sex position is a great way to switch it up.

HOW TO DO IT

The Reverse 69 is a favorite among many couples because it allows both partners to give and experience oral sex simultaneously. In the Reverse 69, the female partner lies on a flat surface on her back, and the male partner straddles her face, facing towards her feet. He then leans down and performs oral sex on her, while simultaneously receiving it.

WHERE TO DO IT

You can do the Reverse 69 on the floor, sofa, bed, reclining chair, outdoors, or anywhere you can both comfortably lie down.

PROPS YOU'LL NEED

None.

DIFFICULTY LEVEL ★☆☆☆☆

HER O-METER ★★★★☆

Reverse 69 is a great way to mix it up and change positions. Just like traditional 69, it's a give-and-take position, so both partners get to experience pleasure at the same time in this position.

HIS O-METER ★★★★☆

He likes Reverse 69 just as much as traditional 69, and maybe even a little more, because he has more control over the thrusting, but this position can also be a little more challenging because he will have to support his weight on his arms, rather than being able to relax and enjoy the sensations.

MAKE IT HOTTER . . .

Hold on tight and roll over together to switch between 69 and Reverse 69, thereby giving both partners equal time on top and bottom.

SIDEWAYS 69

Sideways 69 is the best of both worlds.

HOW TO DO IT

The Sideways-69 oral sex position is a personal favorite because it allows both partners to give and experience oral sex simultaneously, and no one has to be on the top or bottom. In the Sideways 69, both partners are on their sides head to toe. This can be easier on everyone's neck!

WHERE TO DO IT

You can do Sideways 69 on the floor, sofa, bed, reclining chair, outdoors, or anywhere you can both comfortably lie down.

PROPS YOU'LL NEED

None.

DIFFICULTY LEVEL ★☆☆☆☆

HER O-METER ★★★★☆

Sideways 69 is the best of both worlds. Both partners get to relax a little, sit back, and enjoy the pleasure. She particularly likes this one because lying on her side gives her more control over both her pleasure and his level of thrusting.

HIS O-METER ★★★★☆

He will enjoy Sideways 69 for the exact same reasons she does. It's less strenuous and gives him more control over his pleasure because he is free to move around more than he is during traditional 69.

MAKE IT HOTTER . . .

Try adding some flavored oral sex gel to really get the most out of all of the 69 positions.

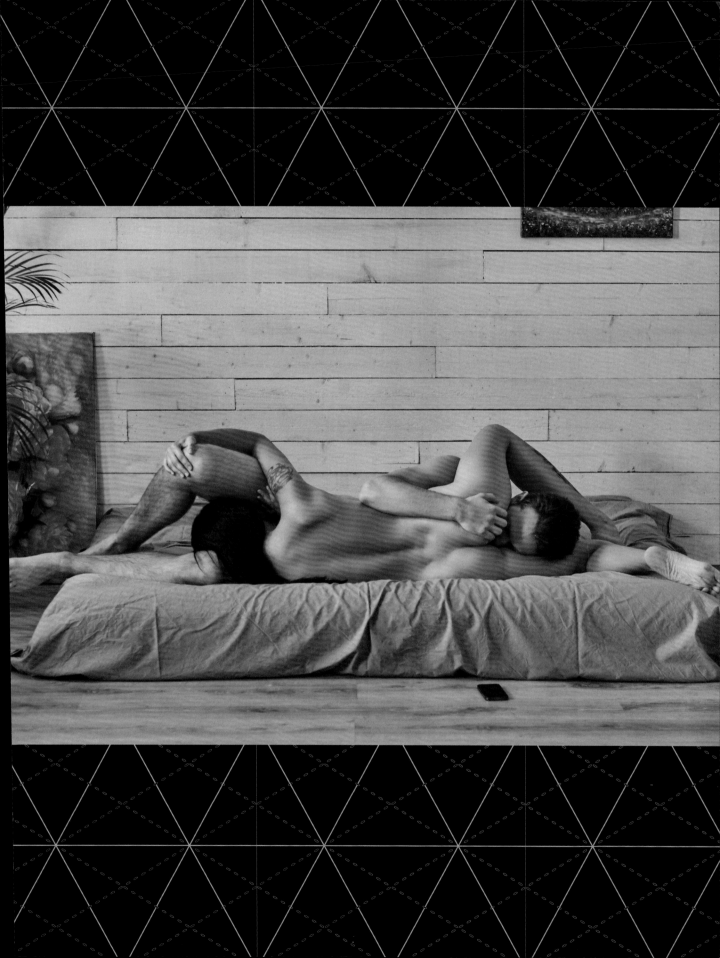

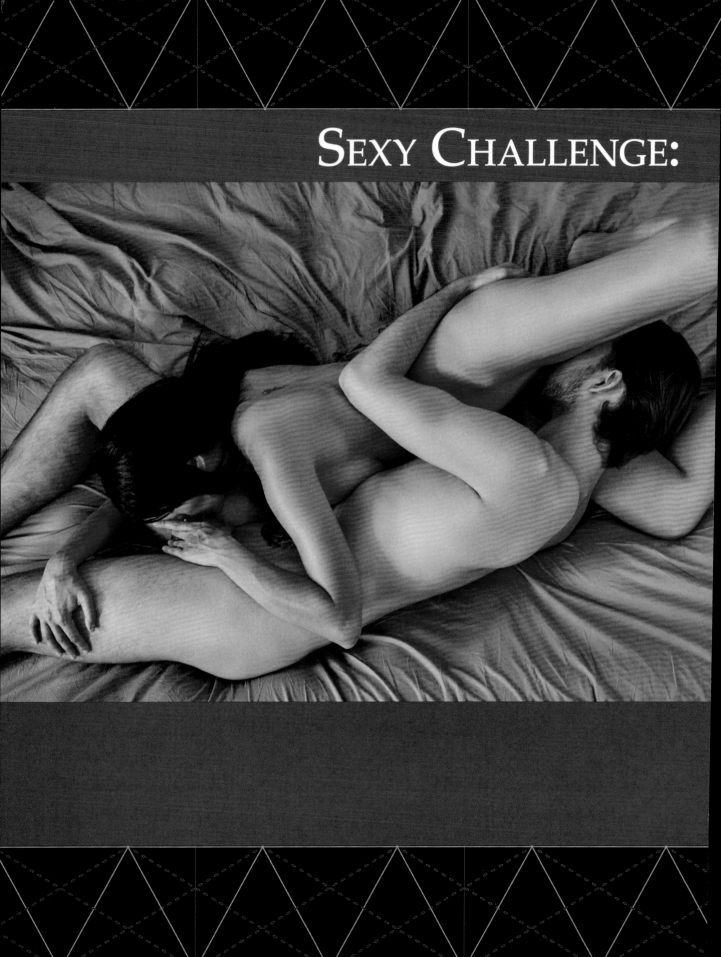

SEXY CHALLENGE:

THE CIRCLE OF PLEASURE

Oral sex is extremely pleasurable, and we all like to sit back and enjoy it, but what if I told you there is a big benefit to doing it at the same time upon each other? We have just come off the 69 sex positions section, but there is more to these positions than just having amazing oral sex. There is a circulation of energy that flows in and out of you as a couple. It you are familiar with tantra, then you know that tantra has a process where you breathe in your partner's breath, and then share yours with them. It is a way of connecting the lovers in a deeper and more connected state. Well, think about how connected lovers can be when we are performing oral sex on each other! Think about the delightful crop circles we mentioned earlier in this book, and how we are now going to circle that sexual energy through both lovers' bodies as they orally pleasure each other.

While performing oral sex on each other at the same time, some interesting things begin to happen. For starters, if you are fluid bonded with your partner, you can consume the love juices that are produced during this process. Many traditions consider the juices that come from the penis and vagina as sacred and powerful. I totally agree with this point that there is a power to consuming the fluids produced by your lover during sexual activity. When you are doing this in the 69 fashion, you are creating a Circle of Pleasure, so that there is a constant flow of all your energies between you and your lover. Think about it when you consume your partner's juices and your partner consumes yours; eventually they work their way through your body and they are shared again with your partner the next time you venture into a 69 situation. In this manner, you get an amazing milkshake of sexual energy.

For the Circle-of-Pleasure Sexy Challenge, I am going to challenge you to perform oral sex on each other in the 69 position to orgasm, each of the next three days. You can mix up the positions in the book to see which ones work the best for you two as a couple. Three days will allow you both to get a good mix of the other person's sexual energy, as well as what happens when some of your own sexual energy is returned to you. I also want you to keep notes on how you feel each of the next mornings. On the third morning, make sure to pay extra special attention to how you feel on that day! It is after the third day that you should not only have consumed the sexual energy of your lover, but also of the combination of the sexual energy of your combined juices. This should be super powerful and maybe the best vitamins you can possibly take. If you want to continue and try to keep this up for a week, you can. Then, you can see how far these amazing feelings can actually reach.

Now, some people might be a little afraid to perform oral sex to orgasm on their partner and consume their juices, if they are not fluid bonded yet. You can still perform this challenge using condoms and dental dams, and there will still be a flow of energy. It still does not give the full effect, but if you are concerned about STDs, or the thought of the experience of consumption doesn't appeal to you, then using prophylactics is a suitable alternative. Some people are concerned with the taste of sexual juices, and you can change the taste based on what you actually eat during the day. Consuming juices is a great way to make your love juices taste different, with pineapple juice being one of the most popular. Also, eating healthy foods is better, so skip the fast-food burgers for a while, and focus on some salad and other healthy alternatives. There are many different thoughts out there on the subject, but if you stick with things that are healthy for you, I am sure it is better. Even drinking and smoking can have a negative effect on taste when it comes to oral sex.

Oral sex is an energy exchange just like passionate kissing. However, oral sex has the power to give a different and more spiritual form of pleasure. While the lips on our face are sensitive and exciting, there is something even more special about experiencing the genitals of our partner in an oral manner. While amazing conversation lights our relationship up, the conversations you have with your partner's genitals in this manner are also a sensational form of conversation with your partner. Expressing this language of oral sexual pleasure is one of the best conversations you can have in your relationship.

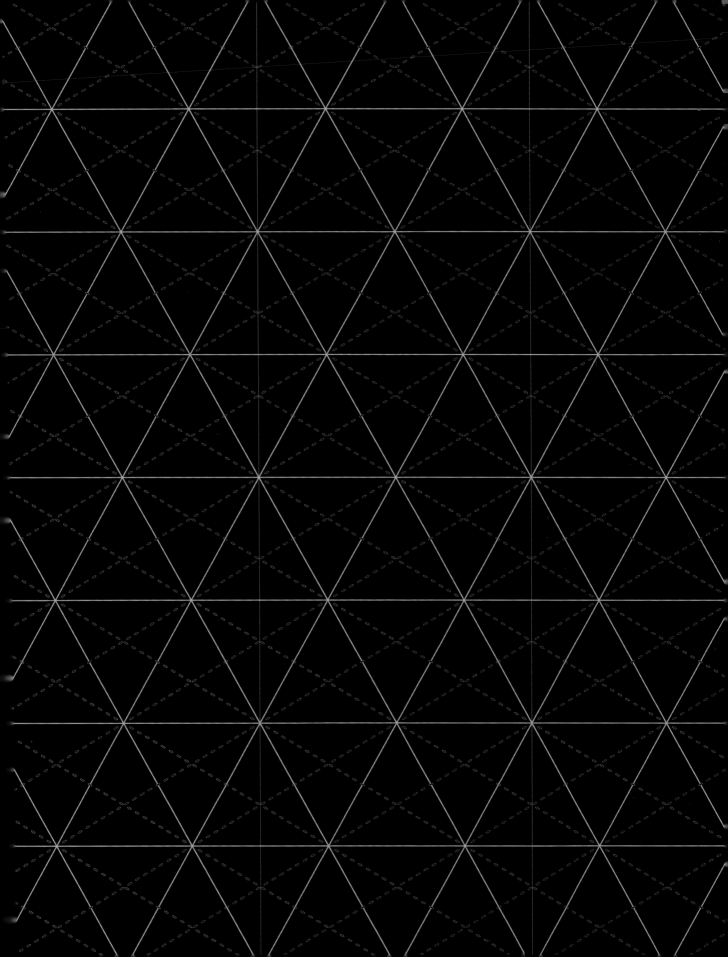

CHAPTER 11: REAR-ENTRY SEX POSITIONS

BASIC REAR ENTRY

This sex position is probably the easiest way to get started with rear entry, apart from Doggy Style (see page 244). When he thrusts, he can stimulate her G-spot in a unique way, and the closer her legs are together, the tighter it feels for him. This is definitely a must try!

HOW TO DO IT

The female partner lies on her stomach and props her upper body up on her elbows. Her legs are slightly spread apart, with her knees bent and feet in the air. The male partner approaches her from behind and drapes his pelvis over her rear, so his penis can enter her vaginal opening from behind. He supports his body weight with his knees and his arms, which are positioned on either side of her upper body. The Basic Rear-Entry sex position can also be used for anal penetration.

WHERE TO DO IT

Rear Entry can be done on the sofa, bed, floor, or any flat surface.

PROPS YOU'LL NEED

A small pillow under her pelvis can raise her bottom to shorten the angle of entry for a man with a shorter penis.

DIFFICULTY LEVEL ★☆☆☆☆

HER O-METER ★★★☆☆

While Basic Rear Entry does provide a unique angle to her G-spot, unless her partner's penis is on the longer side, she's not likely to get as much pleasure from this as she would if she were on top. However, if his penis is big enough, this could stimulate her G-spot in ways she's never felt before!

HIS O-METER ★★★★★

This sex position is one of the better ones for guys. The difference here is that her legs are somewhat closed and her buttocks are tight together, making her vagina feel much tighter to him. This increased friction is enough to send him over the moon!

MAKE IT HOTTER . . .

Since she gets pretty much zero clitoral stimulation in this sex position, and he can't help out because he's supporting his weight on his hands, the female partner can get a lot more pleasure out of this position if she stimulates her clitoris herself, either with her fingers, or a small vibrator like a bullet.

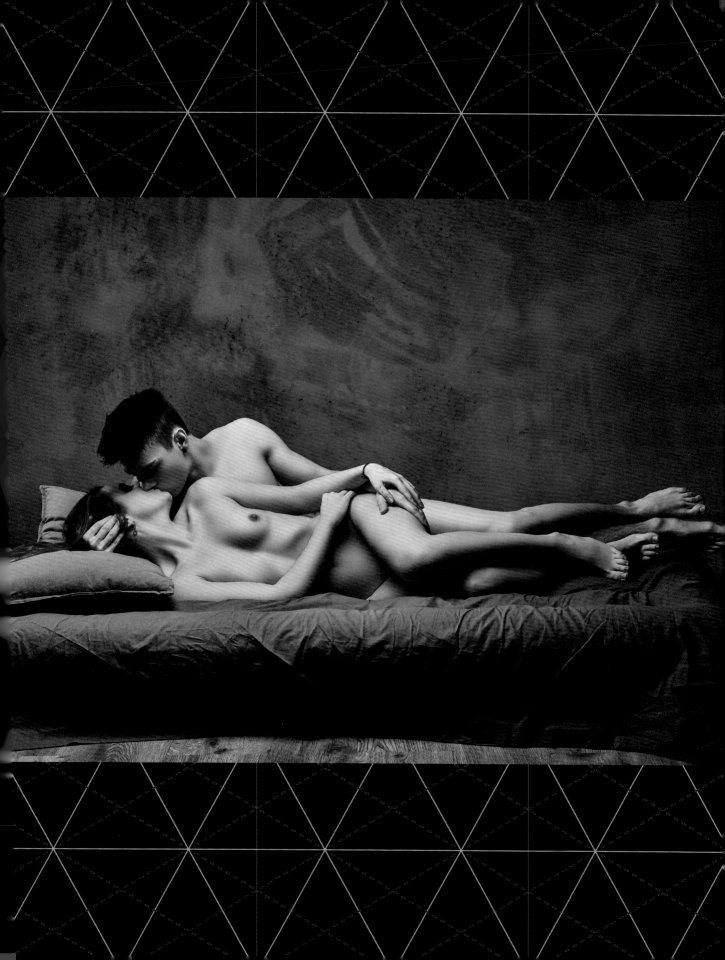

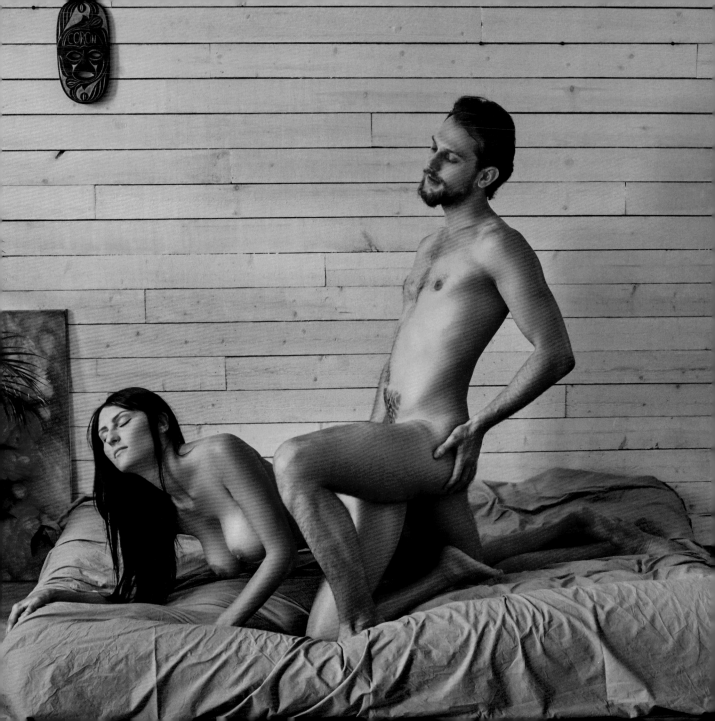

BULLDOG

The Bulldog is a unique take on Doggy Style that requires more leg strength from the male partner, but gives a different penetration angle.

HOW TO DO IT

The female partner assumes the Doggy Style position on all fours (see page 244), and her partner gets behind her. Instead of resting his weight on his knees, he's actually going to crouch down with his feet on the floor or bed, and bend his knees to line up his pelvis with her rear. This can require considerable strength on the male partner's part, especially during thrusting. They'll find that the angle of penetration is quite a bit different from traditional Doggy Style.

WHERE TO DO IT

A flat surface is needed for both partners. She'll need to be on her hands and knees, and he will be crouched down with his weight resting on his feet. It can be done on the bed, but the male partner may be appreciative of the floor, since it will allow him greater stability and balance.

PROPS YOU'LL NEED

If you choose to do the Bulldog on the floor, she'll want something under her knees, like a soft blanket or even a towel to prevent carpet burn.

DIFFICULTY LEVEL ★★★★☆

HER O-METER ★★★☆☆

For women who enjoy deep penetration, G-spot stimulation (without clitoral stimulation), or anal sex, the Bulldog will be right up their alley. It's not as enjoyable for women who need a lot of clitoral stimulation to reach orgasm, but it's still a great spin on Doggy Style when you're looking for something a bit different.

HIS O-METER ★★★☆☆

He likes the Bulldog because the deep penetration feels awesome, but it can be difficult for him to stay crouched in that position for very long, let alone keep up the thrusting action. If he's athletic, it will be easier, but his thighs are definitely going to burn after this one!

MAKE IT HOTTER . . .

If both partners can keep their balance in the Bulldog fairly well, she may be able to reach a hand down and stimulate her clitoris so she gets more out of this position, too.

DOGGY STYLE

Doggy Style is probably the most popular sex position for rear entry, and for good reason! Couples love this position because of how submissive it is for the female partner, and he can watch the action while he thrusts. It's a great position for some good old-fashioned animal sex!

HOW TO DO IT

The female partner gets on all fours with her weight supported on her knees and palms. Her partner approaches her from behind, holding her hips with his hands and supporting his weight with his knees on the floor. This is a great position for rough sex. He has more leverage with his hands on her hips, and can pull her to him or push her away with his arms. It's also an excellent position for deeper penetration.

WHERE TO DO IT

Try Doggy Style on the floor, bed, sofa, the bathtub/shower, or any flat surface with plenty of space.

PROPS YOU'LL NEED

A rolled-up towel or a pillow is almost essential for Doggy Style, unless you're doing it on the bed. It's easy to get carpet burn on your knees if you're having sex on the carpet, or feel uncomfortable on hard surface like a tiled floor or bathtub. Both partners may need some sort of padding under the knees.

DIFFICULTY LEVEL ★☆☆☆☆

HER O-METER ★★★☆☆

Doggy Style is excellent for deep penetration, but not so much for G-spot stimulation. Most men have a penis that angles upwards, which means that during Doggy Style, his penis will "point" towards her lower back (the side of her vagina that her G-spot is not on). However, a woman can really get into Doggy Style if she enjoys rough sex or being dominated in this way. He (or she) can also increase her orgasm potential by stimulating her clitoris.

HIS O-METER ★★★★★

Doggy Style is a favorite among men, simply because many men enjoy being dominant over their partner. After all, the position is called Doggy Style because it mimics what dogs do when a female dog presents herself to a male to be mounted. The act of "presenting" herself in this way makes the woman feel very submissive and the man very dominant, which can be a huge turn on for a man. Not to mention that he gets to stare at her backside the entire time and watch all the action!

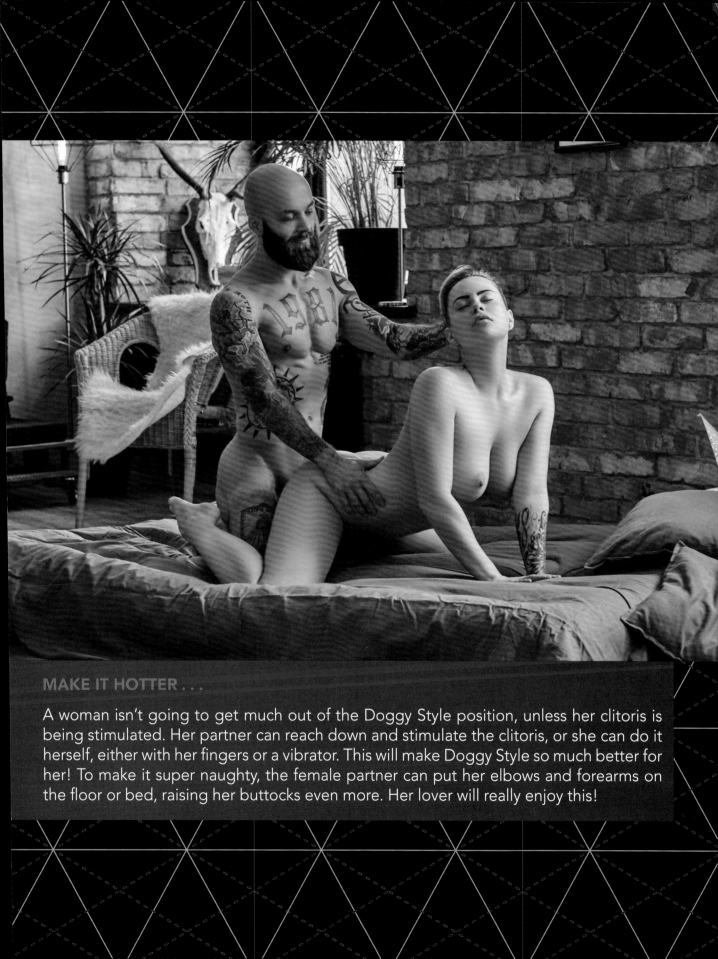

MAKE IT HOTTER . . .

A woman isn't going to get much out of the Doggy Style position, unless her clitoris is being stimulated. Her partner can reach down and stimulate the clitoris, or she can do it herself, either with her fingers or a vibrator. This will make Doggy Style so much better for her! To make it super naughty, the female partner can put her elbows and forearms on the floor or bed, raising her buttocks even more. Her lover will really enjoy this!

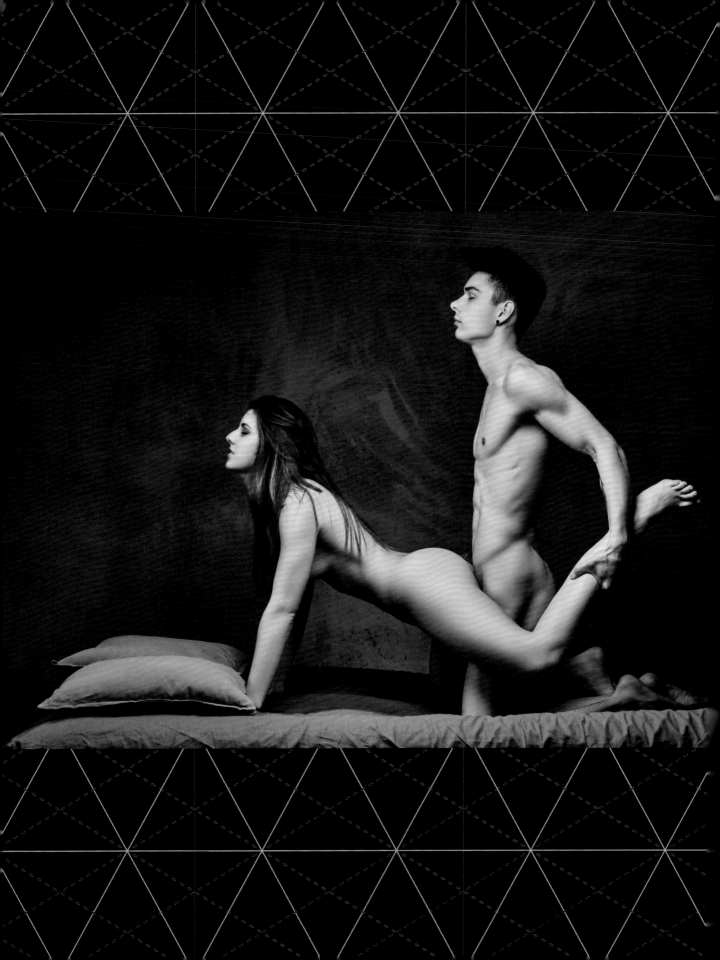

FIRE HYDRANT

The Fire Hydrant is a fun rear-entry position that will bring out the animal in both partners! It's easy to do, but also super sexy. It's a simple variation on Doggy Style that mimics a dog "peeing" on a fire hydrant, hence the name. The position creates deeper penetration and gives both partners access to her clitoris.

HOW TO DO IT

The Fire Hydrant starts in the traditional Doggy Style position, with her on all fours and him entering her from behind. Then she simply lifts up one of her legs and hooks it around his hip and buttock.

WHERE TO DO IT

The Fire Hydrant can be done anywhere you would do Doggy Style!

PROPS YOU'LL NEED

If you're not having sex on a bed or other comfortable surface, a soft blanket will protect the knees of both partners.

DIFFICULTY LEVEL ★☆☆☆☆

HER O-METER ★★★☆☆

While the Fire Hydrant sex position doesn't afford a lot of clitoral stimulation, it does provide great access to the G-spot, and even the A-spot with penetration being so deep.

HIS O-METER ★★★★☆

He loves the animalistic feel of this sex position, in which he can pull her towards him as he thrusts. He'll really like her leg hooked around him, and he can even reach down and stimulate her clitoris and labia with his hands as he gets his groove on.

MAKE IT HOTTER . . .

If you have a large mirror, set it on the floor and have sex on it. The Fire Hydrant opens her legs up for a very nice, and (ahem) not modest, view of the action!

FROG LEAP

The Frog-Leap sex position is a super naughty twist on Doggy Style that gives him full access to her and facilitates super-deep penetration. It's hot!

HOW TO DO IT

The Frog Leap gets its name from the way the female partner is positioned for thrusting. She is on her hands and feet with her knees bent, as though she were getting ready to play the childhood game of leapfrogs. The male partner sits on his knees behind her like in traditional Doggy Style, and holds onto her hips while he thrusts. This creates deep penetration and new sensations for both partners!

WHERE TO DO IT

The floor is probably the best place for the Frog Leap, simply because the female partner needs a hard surface without a lot of give to it to maintain her balance.

PROPS YOU'LL NEED

He might want a pillow for his knees, and a large soft blanket is always nice when you're dealing with carpet (although carpet burns can lead to interesting conversations the next day at work).

DIFFICULTY LEVEL ★☆☆☆☆

HER O-METER ★☆☆☆☆

The Frog Leap is an awkward one for her to get into and stay in, unless she's on the thinner side and has a lot of strength in her legs.

HIS O-METER ★★★★☆

He really enjoys the control he has in the Frog Leap, and it's comfortable for him because he isn't doing anything differently than he normally does in the Doggy-Style sex position. He will also enjoy the view, especially if he prefers butts to breasts, or likes anal play at all.

MAKE IT HOTTER . . .

Do it on the bed and have her grab on to the headboard, or on a landing with a railing that she can grab on to. This will help support her and make this move super hot!

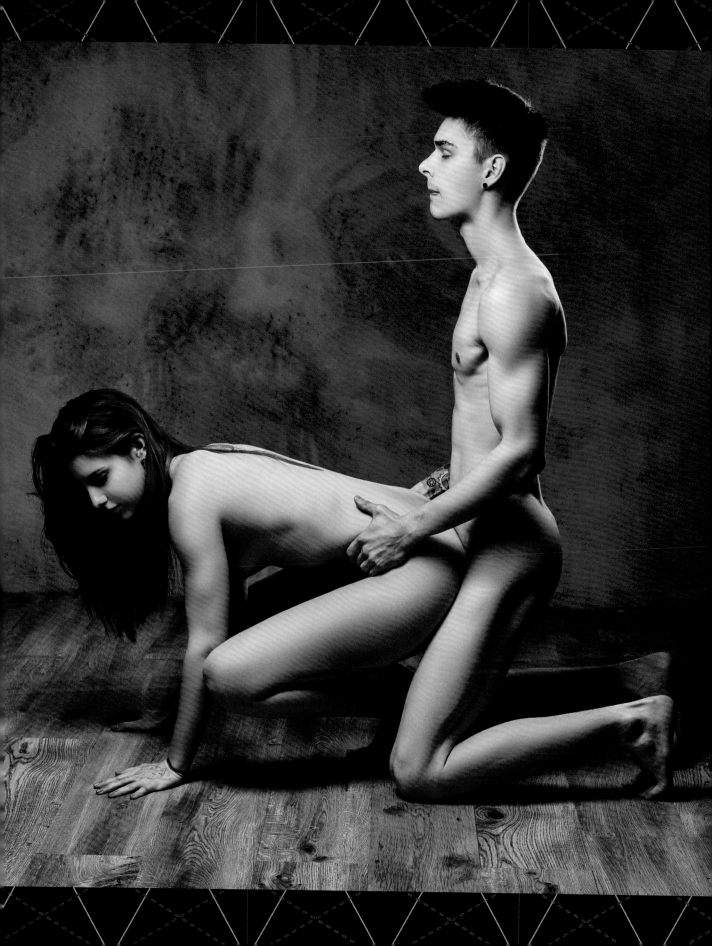

GRASSHOPPER

While the Grasshopper causes the penis to bend in an awkward way, this position can be super erotic for the flexible man. If you like exotic sex positions, the Grasshopper is definitely one you'll want to try at least want once.

HOW TO DO IT

The female partner lies on a flat surface on her stomach, with her legs stretched out. She can either lift her torso up on her arms, or she can lie her head down on a pillow if she likes. The male partner does all the work here, like in the Reverse Jockey position (see page 33), but it's a little more challenging for him because the angle of penetration causes the penis to bend in an unnatural way. He will sit on the back of her thighs, just under her buttocks, and point his penis downward to enter her. His legs are open, with each foot is on either side of his lover's waist, and his hands are behind him and by her feet, supporting his weight. He'll want to be very erect before attempting the Grasshopper; a soft or semi-soft penis isn't going to penetrate very well in this position.

WARNING: Go slow when trying this, and if the angle of penetration is at all uncomfortable or painful, stop immediately! Some men just don't have the flexibility to do the Grasshopper and that's perfectly OK. You don't want to end up with a penile fracture just to say you tried this position.

WHERE TO DO IT

Although this can be done on any flat surface with enough space, the bed is probably a better bet than the floor for the Grasshopper. Since you're so focused on the angle of penetration, and just how you're going to get in this position, you don't want to add any logistical worries.

PROPS YOU'LL NEED

She may want a pillow for her head if she's not holding her torso up with her arms, but it's not necessary.

DIFFICULTY LEVEL ★★★★★

HER O-METER ★☆☆☆☆

He's not grinding up against her clitoris in the Grasshopper, and because his penis is at an awkward angle, she won't get much G-spot stimulation either. This is, however, a comfortable position for her while her lover works on his thrusting technique.

HIS O-METER ★☆☆☆☆

The odd angle of the penis in this position won't be comfortable for many men, and the thrusting action is going to be hard to figure out too. The Grasshopper is really just a novelty position to try.

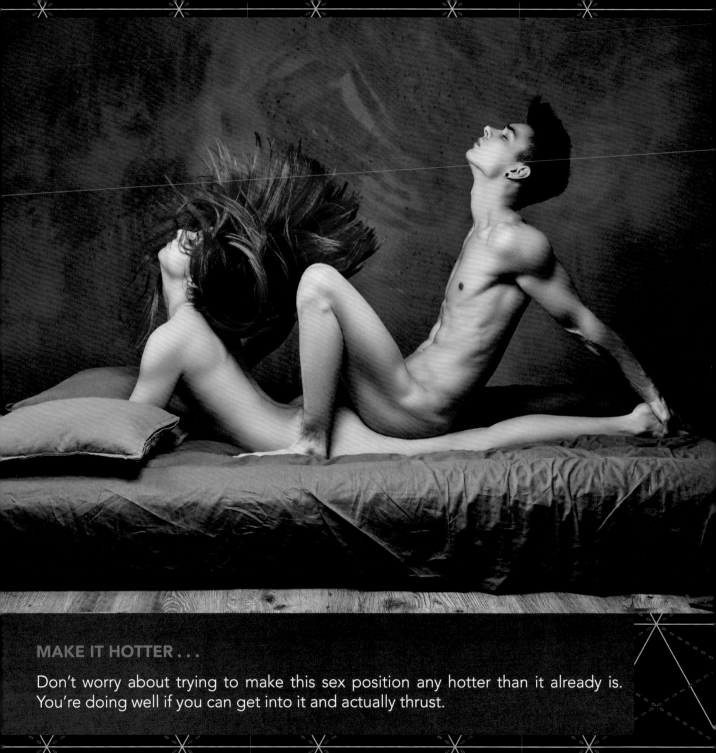

MAKE IT HOTTER . . .

Don't worry about trying to make this sex position any hotter than it already is. You're doing well if you can get into it and actually thrust.

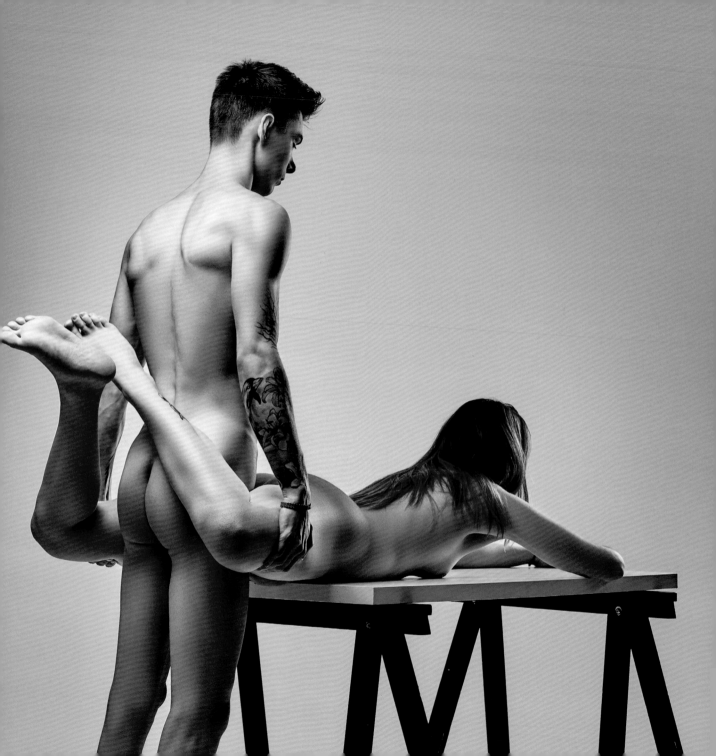

LIFE RAFT

The Life Raft is a fairly easy, but exciting, twist on Doggy Style, and is especially fun for the male partner. This is definitely a must try, whether it becomes one of your favorites or not.

HOW TO DO IT

The female partner lays on the edge of table, desk, or bed on her belly, with her knees bent and spread a little farther than shoulder width apart. The male partner comes up behind her, lifting her knees, and hitching them up around his hips where he can penetrate her. This may be easier to do if he penetrates first, and then wraps her legs around him. She'll continue to keep her legs wrapped around him while he thrusts.

WHERE TO DO IT

The Life-Raft sex position requires a bed or other surface like a desk or table that is approximately hip height.

PROPS YOU'LL NEED

A blanket or thick towel is recommended if a desk or table is used. It will make this position more comfortable for her.

DIFFICULTY LEVEL ★☆☆☆☆

HER O-METER ★☆☆☆☆

The Life Raft is a position that she's not going to get much from in and of itself. She can reach her hands down and stimulate her clitoris for more pleasure during intercourse, but unless she really digs rear-entry or anal sex, this is not going to be at the top of her list. It is, however, fairly comfortable for her since her lover is supporting her legs, so most women don't have a problem giving this one a try for their partners.

HIS O-METER ★★★☆☆

This is a great sex position for "butt guys," but it may get a little tiresome for him to hold her legs up and thrust at the same time. The Life Raft is still a fun one to try, because he really may like the angle of penetration and how she's spread out just for him!

MAKE IT HOTTER . . .

Add a pillow or rolled-up towel under her hips to enhance the angle of penetration.

TURTLE

The Turtle is an easy twist on Doggy Style that will add some spice to an old favorite. He really enjoys how submissive she is here, and how in control he is.

HOW TO DO IT

The female partner rests her weight on her knees and folds over, putting her forehead as close to her knees as possible. Her breasts will be resting against the top of her thighs and she'll look almost like a turtle, hence the name. The male partner enters her from behind, with his legs spread on either side of her, almost like traditional Doggy Style. It's an easy position to get into and stay in, and it's a simple twist on an old favorite if you're looking for something new to do.

WHERE TO DO IT

A flat surface with a fair amount of space, such as on the floor or in the bed. The sofa or the back seat of a car won't work very well for the Turtle because of the way the male partner needs to spread his legs.

PROPS YOU'LL NEED

She may want a pillow under her knees, or a blanket if you're on the floor.

DIFFICULTY LEVEL ★☆☆☆☆

HER O-METER ★☆☆☆☆

Even though there's some G-spot stimulation in the Turtle, this probably won't be a favorite sex position for her. Without clitoral stimulation or even face-to-face contact, it's going to be very difficult for her to actually reach orgasm here.

HIS O-METER ★★★☆☆

Although this is a fun twist on Doggy Style for him and he enjoys how submissive she is in the Turtle, there's not much for him to look at here besides his lover's back. This is a fun one to try, but it's not going to be one of his all-time favorites either.

MAKE IT HOTTER . . .

If you're into BDSM at all, this can be a fun sex position to incorporate some bondage into. Her hands can be bound to her ankles in this position for an ultra-submissive variation.

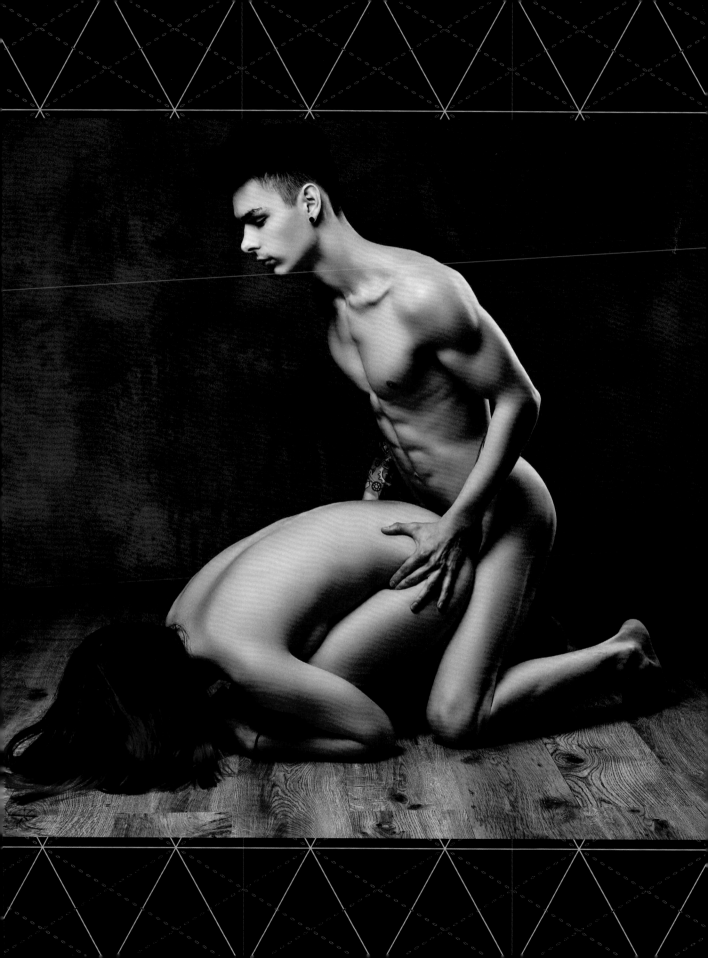

YOGA MASTER

For the athletic man, the Yoga Master is an exotic rear-entry position that is a perfect fit for the super adventurous couple.

HOW TO DO IT

The female partner lies on the bed on her stomach, with her hips at the edge of the bed and her torso hanging off. She rests her hands and head on the floor, while he mounts her from behind on the bed. Her legs are closed and straight, and his are as well, lining up with her legs. He penetrates her from behind and uses his hands to arch his back up (almost like the Upward Facing Dog yoga move) and thrust. This is a fairly difficult position to do, but can be highly rewarding for the couple who enjoys very exotic sex.

WHERE TO DO IT

This is a sex position to use on the bed. You'll be using the edge of it, but it's just not one you can do anywhere else.

PROPS YOU'LL NEED

She will definitely want a pillow if her head is on the floor!

DIFFICULTY LEVEL ★★★★★

HER O-METER ★☆☆☆☆

She may not like the Yoga Master as much as he does, simply because there is very little in it for her unless she really enjoys rear-entry or anal penetration. Her clitoris is well hidden, and neither partner can really reach it to stimulate it. Also, because of the position of both his legs and hers, he can't penetrate her very deeply, especially if his penis is smaller. However, if she enjoys exotic positions, she will like how different this one is from others.

HIS O-METER ★★★☆☆

Although the Yoga Master is strenuous on him, he'll like how unique and exotic it is, if he's adventurous. The flexible man with strong arms will likely not have much difficulty with this position, but getting the thrusting action down pat can be a bit difficult.

MAKE IT HOTTER . . .

Practice this one by starting with basic Rear Entry, using a Liberator Wedge. He can also achieve a similar effect by standing and bending her over the back of a sofa or chair.

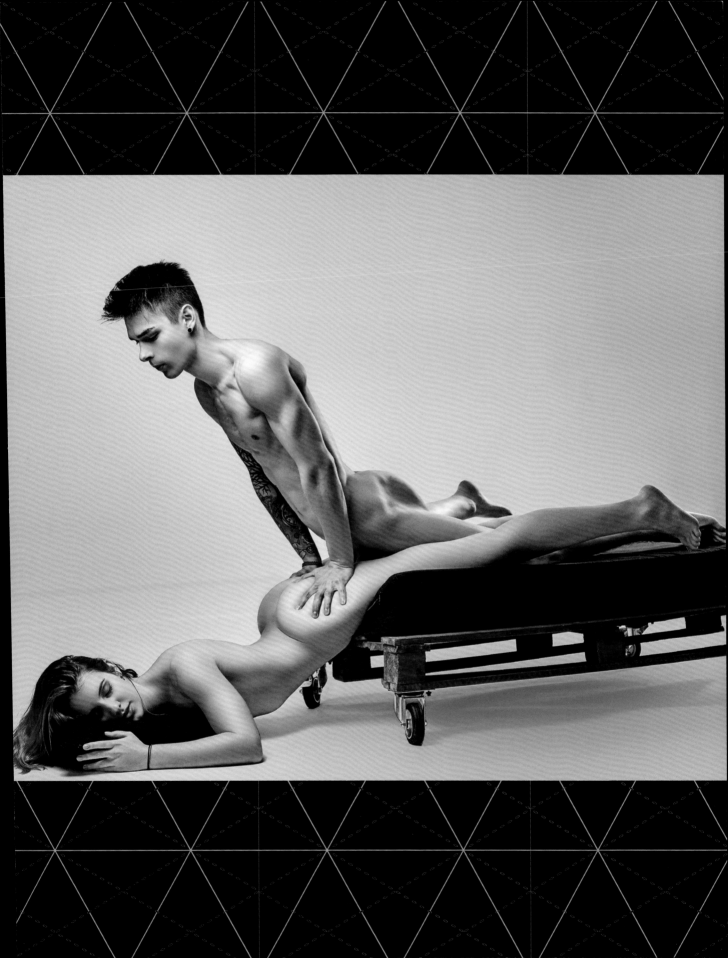

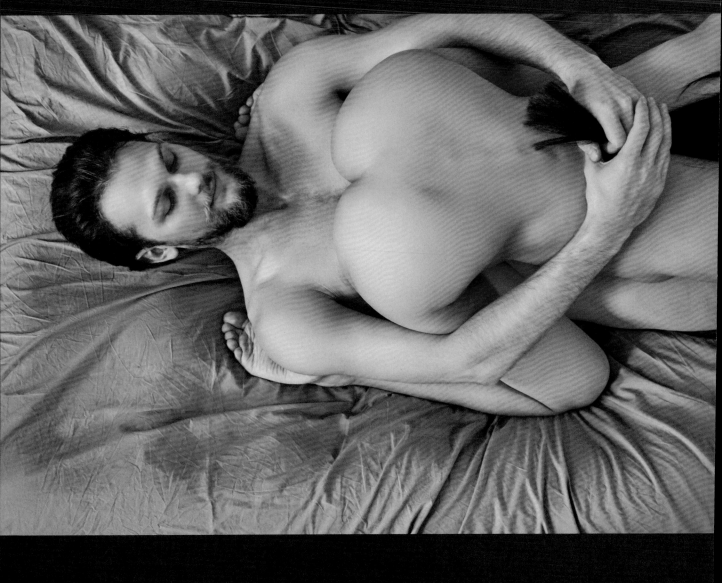

SEXY CHALLENGE:

Rear-entry positions are the most primal and animalistic positions that sex has to offer, in my opinion. While these rear-entry positions feel very natural and basic, they also allow both partners the options of connecting to something much different than all the other sexual positions. Rear-entry positions can be aggressively engaged by both partners allowing for a more enthusiastic experience together. But the thing this Sexy Challenge of a Vision Quest wants to focus on is the fact that both partners are facing the same direction. In essence, both partners are facing ahead, looking toward what is coming towards them. If you think of the sexual experience as a journey or a travel, then you need to see what is ahead of you, and together you can witness not only the forceful pleasure of the rear-entry position, but what also is coming into your life based on your sexual energy.

So, we have talked in previous chapters about being able to see sexual energy. In this Sexy Challenge of the Vision Quest, both partners are going to be able to be in the driver's seat. As mentioned earlier, both partners will be facing the same way, and both partners can control the aggressive thrusting. The man can be thrusting his penis into the woman, and the woman can also be thrusting herself back to take more of the penis in an aggressive manner. The Doggy-Style position is great for this Vision Quest and is one of the most basic rear-entry positions. With the man thrusting forward and the woman thrusting back, we get something amazing happening in the middle: a portal is being opened that will allow for experiences and visions to come out into play. Think of the Big Bang that created our universe and how it released items that would later become planets, stars, asteroids, etc., making our universe its own canvas of amazing beauty. So, with each thrust that comes together, we are creating that same Big Bang, just on a little smaller scale.

Each thrust will release items for our Vision Quest. Now, you have to understand that each vision might not be able to be seen with your naked eye, it might pop into your mind, or it might come visit you later in a dream. The point is, in our Sexy Challenge Vision Quest, we need to be open to collecting all the images or feelings we experience. The more aggressive and pleasurable the thrusting, the more we force out these visions and allow them to flow. It is also a great idea to sync your thrusting, so that you are meeting together at the Big-Bang place, as that will give you both the most satisfaction and ability to experience the Vision Quest. Now, the thrusting can become quick and rapid, especially as one partner is nearing climax, so be prepared because each thrust can force out visions from the portal between the two of you. From time to time, you might want to slow down and enjoy some slower thrusting to see if it allows you more of a chance to experience the visions.

Most of the Vision Quest will be able to be seen while you are looking in front of you, as if you had a screen in front of you. However, there are times you might witness something in different directions. Maybe you will catch something out of the corner of your eye, or maybe you will lower your head to achieve a different angle of penetration and have to turn your head to the side. No matter which way you will look, if you open yourself up, you will start to see the Vision Quest unfold. I actually suggest at some point during the rear-entry position that you try closing your eyes; even if you have your eyes closed, your mind will assist you and show you the images. Start to pay even more attention to the feelings and your scenes as you near climax, for at that moment, there will be a flood of visions shared between the two of you. While it is difficult to concentrate at this moment, if you can pay attention, you can you will be treated to an otherworldly delight.

All of the rear-entry positions in this book will allow you to experience your dimensional visions, as you spend the evening connected to each other in the most natural way. Yet you might find one position that takes it to a higher level for you, so please try out all the rear-entry positions and see what works the best for you. You can also help to stimulate your partner by helping them to get some different Visions to pop into their head. From behind, you can slap their ass, or reach up and pull on your partner's nipples, and you can lean forward and bite your partners back, not to mention use other toys or devices to turn up the volume of pleasure. The partner in front can easily change the angle of penetration; they can also reach under and fondle, squeeze, or tug on the scrotum of the one thrusting, and they can grab a toy or two and stimulate areas of their partner's body. The possibilities are endless, and the visions will be too.

Some variations you might want to try are to do this in complete darkness—it is sometimes easier to see the visions without any lighting of any sort that could distract from the Vision Quest. Another great idea would be to do this facing into a mirror, as mirrors have many magical qualities, and could bring visions happening behind you to the front. If you are brave enough, you might even film the event and watch it together later. You might be surprised at what you might see going on in the room while you are getting busy and focused on pleasure. Remember, you are creating sexual energy, and that energy is wild and alive and it could be doing all sorts of things in the room.

Lastly, I want to remind you to pay attention that after the fact, during what I call the valley, your body is returning to its normal state. Your breathing is returning to normal and you are basking in the pleasure you have just had; it is a great time for visions to be seen. You can also experience your Vision Quest during your sleep cycle after all is said and done. So, prepare yourself to accept any amazing dreams as part of your Vision Quest. Remember that with any Sexy Challenge, you might have to practice a little bit to master it. So, if your first time isn't fireworks, don't be alarmed. As you open yourself up more and more, the visions will appear and you will be very happy.

Chapter 12: BDSM for Lovers

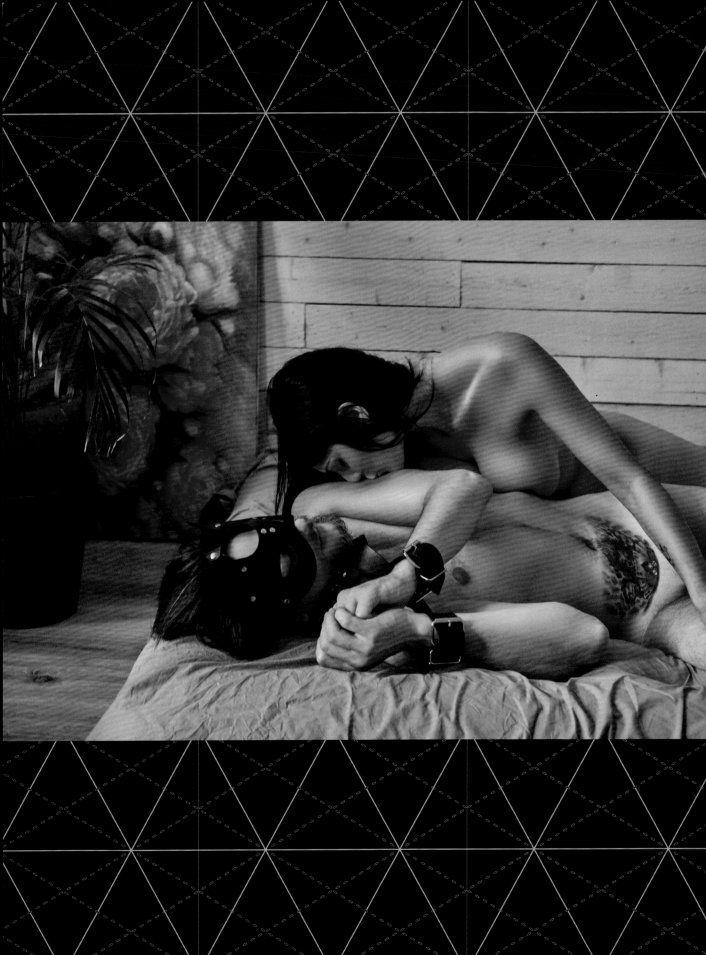

BOUNDARIES AND LIMITS (HOW TO)

As we all know, half the fun in BDSM is finding out where our boundaries are and giving them a little push.

While you might not think that you like sensation play—things that tweak your senses like heat, ice, or even tickling— but why not push that boundary and give it a try? You might be surprised . . . Gently pushing our preconceived boundaries can result in a whole new level of intimacy and ecstasy!

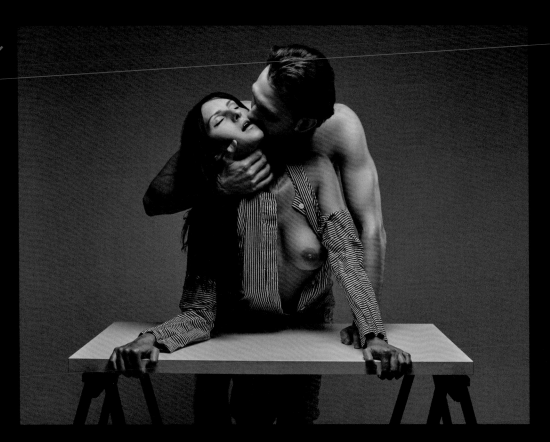

But how can you push boundaries in a way that is both physically and emotionally safe?

Let's talk briefly about hard limits and soft limits. A hard limit is something that you are not willing to do under any circumstances. A soft limit is something that you may be willing to do with the right person and only under certain conditions.

See the end of this chapter for a sample BDSM checklist to help you and your partner better understand each of your boundaries and limits. Take some time to complete the checklist and talk about the topics that you want to explore together.

266 bdsm for lovers

When you do start experimenting and pushing, take it slow, and after each play session talk about what worked, what didn't, and where your play should go next time. I also recommend implementing the standard color system during your play sessions:

Green = Keep going. I love what you're doing.

Yellow = This is a little intense for me, let's slow down or take a break, then continue.

Red = STOP immediately and do not continue. This is too much and the session needs to end.

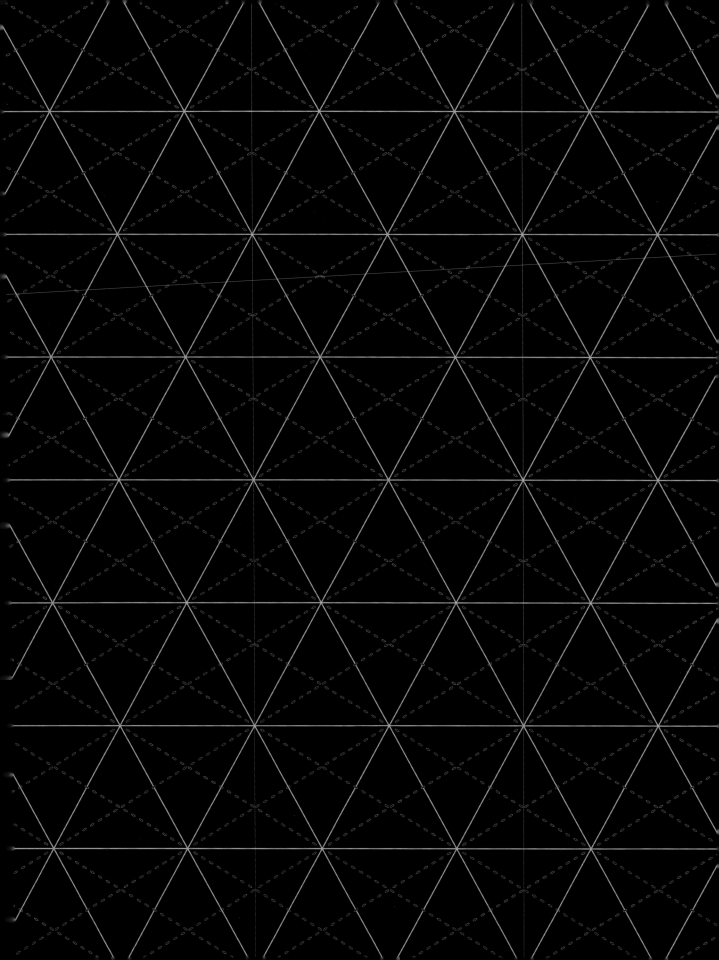

ADVENTURE CHECKLIST

The following is an adaptation of the original "Adventure Checklist" from Dr. Michael Harris (https://drmichaelharris.com/erotic-hypnosis/).

This checklist is not gender specific or orientation specific, so adjust where necessary. Many people wish to be sexually adventurous, but really don't know where to begin. This checklist is by no means exhaustive, but it will serve as a catalyst for discovery and conversation. It has been simplified for the sake of brevity, as the original Adventure Checklist is incredibly detailed. I highly recommend that you go to his website and complete the full checklist as time allows. If you have any questions or would like to know more about the checklist or erotic hypnosis, please contact him directly.

Please rate your interest of each topic from 0 to 5, and also indicate whether you are interested in giving or receiving or both (G, R, B).

Level of interests from 0 to 5:

0 = I will not do/try that item under ANY circumstances (a hard limit).

1 = No desire, don't like, but will if it's really important to my partner (a soft limit).

2 = Willing to do/try, but has no special appeal.

3 = Usually LIKE doing (willing to try), on an occasional basis.

4 = LIKE doing and would like it on a regular basis. (Want to try.)

5 = WILD TURN-ON, I would like it as often as possible. (REALLY want to try.)

ACTIVITY	INTEREST (0-5)	GIVE/RECEIVE/BOTH
Anal sex		
Anal role play (puppy/pony/kitten or other)		
Biting		
Blindfolds		
Bondage (light/medium/ heavy; metal/leather/rope)		
Breath control and/or choking		
Cells/closets (any type of confinement)		
Chastity belts or Cock caging		
Clothespins		
Clothing—slutty (public/private)		
Clothing (rubber/latex/leather)		
Collars (private/public/symbolic)		
Cuckold (public/private)		
Cuffs (leather/metal)		
Cunnilingus (Oral sex for her)		
Dildo or vibrators (vaginal or anal)		
Double or triple penetration		
Edging (masturbation without orgasm)		
Electricity		
Enforced chastity		
Erotic dance (for audience/private)		

ACTIVITY	INTEREST (0-5)	GIVE/RECEIVE/BOTH
Exhibitionism (being watched)		
Voyeurism (watching others)		
Face or mouth fucking		
Face slapping		
Fantasy abandonment		
Fantasy rape		
Fisting (vaginal or anal)		
Flogging		
Following orders		
Food play		
Full heads hoods		
Gags (ball/cloth/phallus/ rubber/tape)		
Golden showers		
Hair pulling		
Hand jobs (getting or giving, man or woman)		
Harems (real or fantasy)		
Hot oils or wax		
Humiliation (pubic/private)		
Lingerie (public/private)		
Masturbation (public/private)		
Medical scenes (giving or receiving)		
Mummification or saran wrapping (face/head/body)		
Nipple torture (clamps)		
Outdoor sex		
Pain (mild/medium/severe)		
Pegging		

ACTIVITY	INTEREST (0-5)	GIVE/RECEIVE/BOTH
Phone sex		
Public exposure or nudity		
Pussy or cock whipping		
Rimming (ass licking)		
Scenes (photo/video taped)		
Sex (F/F or M/M)		
Slavery (fantasy/real)		
Spanking		
Spreader bars		
Strap-on dildo (penetration/sucking/wearing)		
Submission (submitting to partner/others)		
Swallowing (semen/urine)		

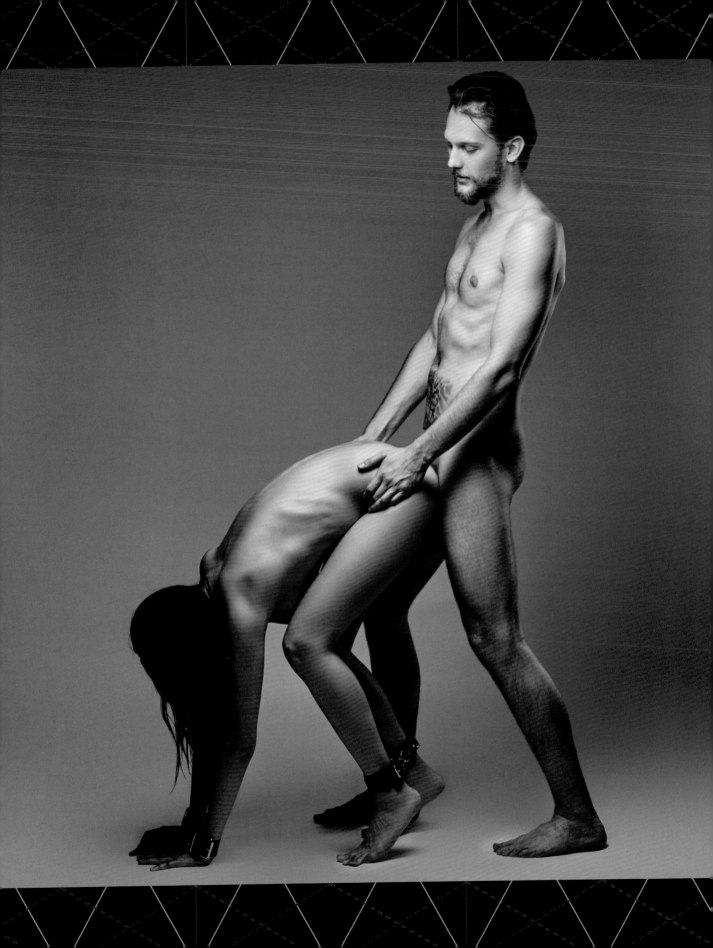

Bent Over and Bound

He is in control as she bends over and he has his way with her, creating deep penetration in a standing sex position.

HOW TO DO IT

Bent Over and Bound is relatively easy to do, and provides for very deep penetration. While she doesn't have to be bound to get intense enjoyment out of this position, you can use rope, leather cuffs, and even add in a spreader bar to tie her wrists and legs together, apart, or to an object, such as the bed or table leg. The variations of this position are limited only by your imagination!

The male partner stands with his legs slightly spread, and his partner stands in front of him with her back to him. She bends over as far as she can, with her legs as straight as possible. This is not always easy if a woman isn't flexible, so a slight bend in the knees is OK here, or she can place her hands on a low stool or ottoman. He will hold her hips to facilitate thrusting, going slowly at first because penetration can be quite deep in this sex position.

For couples who are very different in height, have the taller partner spread his or her legs apart until your hips are at approximately the same height. Doing this on the stairs can also help with a height difference. Just make sure there is something to hold on to!

WHERE TO DO IT

You don't need much space since both partners are standing, and you don't really need to be that undressed to do it either; both partners can simply drop their drawers for a dirty quickie! Try doing this in the department store dressing room or in the bathroom at a party. You may have to forgo the "bound" aspect, but it will still be very hot!

PROPS YOU'LL NEED

Optional leather or metal cuffs, rope, silk ties, spreader bar.

DIFFICULTY LEVEL ★☆☆☆☆

HER O-METER ★☆☆☆☆

Bent Over and Bound may be a bit difficult for her if her legs aren't very flexible. However, some simple stretching can make it easier for her to bend down to reach her toes. Although this sex position doesn't afford any clitoral stimulation, women who enjoy feeling submissive and vulnerable during sex—as well as women who enjoy very deep penetration—will add this sex position to their list of favorites.

HIS O-METER ★★★★★

He loves the feeling of control and dominance he has over his lover in the Bent Over and Bound. He loves the view, and he loves the deep penetration. This position also allows him to wrap his hands around her hips and pull her into his thrusts for even more control. There's simply nothing about this sex position that he doesn't like!

MAKE IT HOTTER . . .

Bent Over and Bound is a great one to use in the midst of a domination-submissive role play scenario in which the male partner is dominant. He can thrust deeply if she's comfortable with that, he can talk dirty, and he can even give her a few spankings for being naughty as he's having sex with her!

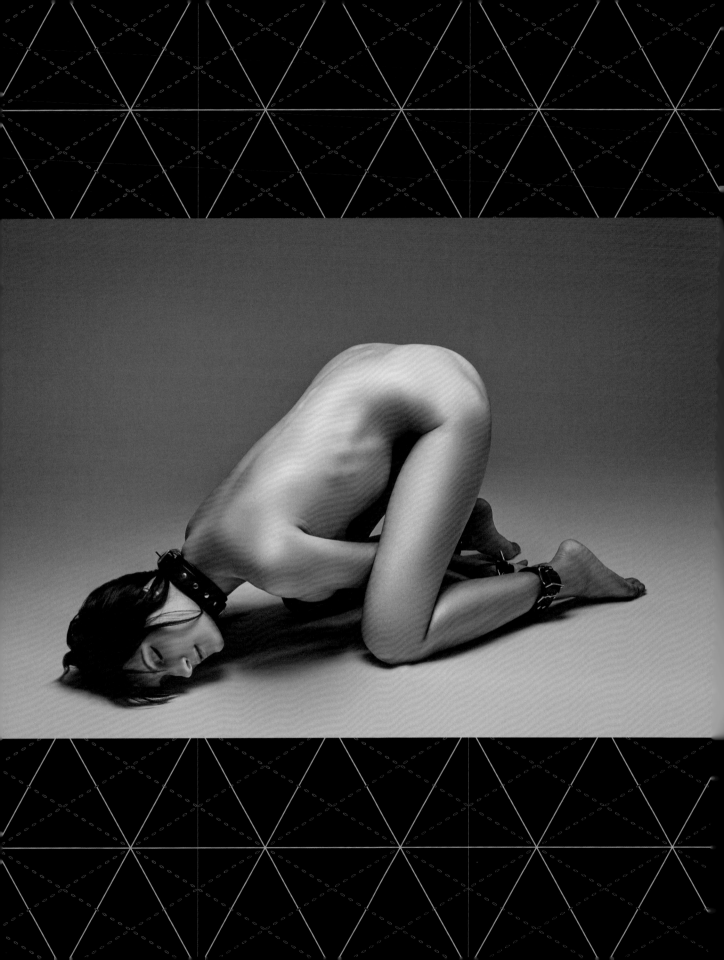

FROG LEAP BOUND

The Frog-Leap sex position is a super naughty twist on Doggy Style that gives him full access to her and facilitates super-deep penetration. Frog Leap Bound takes it to a whole other level!

HOW TO DO IT

The Frog Leap Bound takes the standard Frog Leap and rotates her down to rest on her face. Plus, she is bound at the ankle and wrists, with her wrist restraints attached to the ankle restraints. The male partner sits on his knees behind her like in traditional Doggy Style, and holds onto her hips while he thrusts. This is truly one of the hottest positions in the entire book!

WHERE TO DO IT

The floor or bed works best for this position, but just about any firm flat surface will work.

PROPS YOU'LL NEED

You'll need some ankle and wrist restraints. Leather or cloth will be the most comfortable in this position.

DIFFICULTY LEVEL ★☆☆☆☆

HER O-METER ★★★★☆

If she likes Doggy Style and enjoys being submissive, she will love this position. All she has to do is lay there and enjoy the erotic pleasure of her partner truly "taking" her.

HIS O-METER ★★★★★

This will be one of his all-time favorites. What's not to love about this position? However, if he is super tall, he may need to put her on the bed and stand next to the bed so that this becomes a standing position for him.

MAKE IT HOTTER . . .

Make this one hotter by starting out with her on her knees. Kneeling is a very submissive posture, and he can have his way with her for a few minutes using whatever implements of pleasure they both enjoy. Then push her down and penetrate her from behind.

BOSS'S CHAIR

If he wants to be in control of oral sex, this is one of the best positions to go with! It's a very sexy form of submission on the female partner's part, and is also an easy position for her to give head in. With reduced neck cramps, she'll have lots of stamina here.

HOW TO DO IT

The Boss's-Chair position is popular simply because it's easy to do and can be done almost anywhere a man can sit! The male partner sits on the edge of the sofa or bed, or in a chair, and the female partner kneels in front of him, leaning down to give him oral sex. It's an excellent position for him to be able to watch all of the action!

WHERE TO DO IT

The ideal location for this one is obviously his office chair. This one is particularly hot when performed with her under his office desk!

PROPS YOU'LL NEED

Add a pillow for her knees or buttocks (if she prefers to sit).

DIFFICULTY LEVEL ★☆☆☆☆

HER O-METER ★☆☆☆☆

Let's face it, this one is all for him and that's perfectly OK. She can take pleasure in his pleasure.

HIS O-METER ★★★★★

This is another oral sex position that guys love. But then again, there aren't that many positions that guys won't like if they're getting a blow-job. What men love most about this position is that they're comfortable, but they're also sitting up so they have a good view of what she's doing. Ladies, keep long hair tied back so he can actually see you suck him off. If your hair is all around your face, he might think it's Cousin It giving him head instead.

MAKE IT HOTTER...

Ladies, let your man hold a camera (or he can use his camera phone) to video the blowjob. The Boss's-Chair oral sex position makes for excellent POV (point-of-view) style porn for him to fantasize about you later. Make sure to look up at him with those sexy eyes!

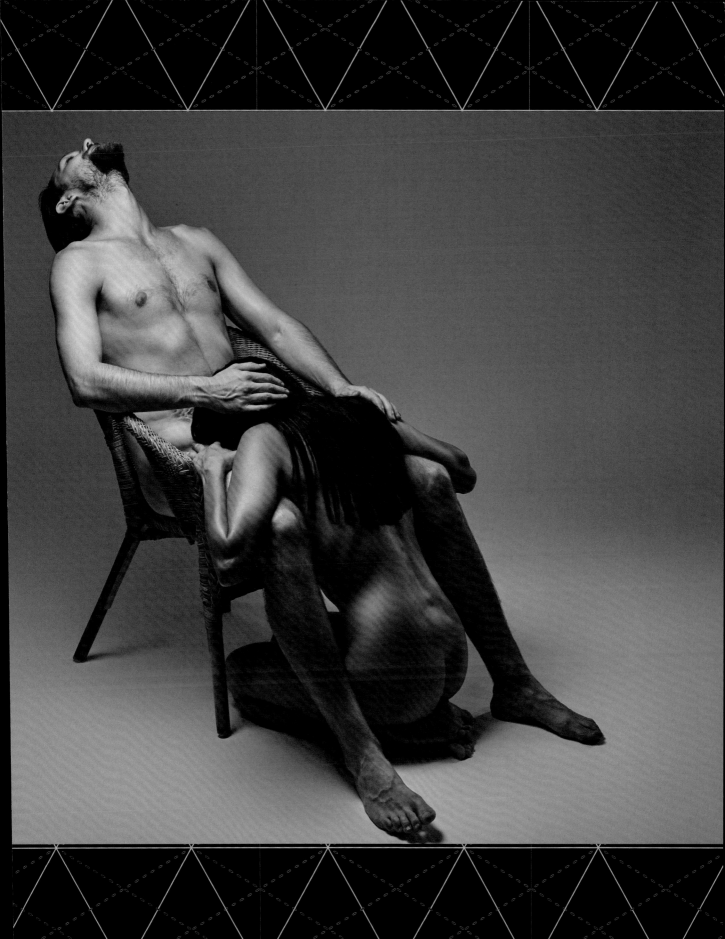

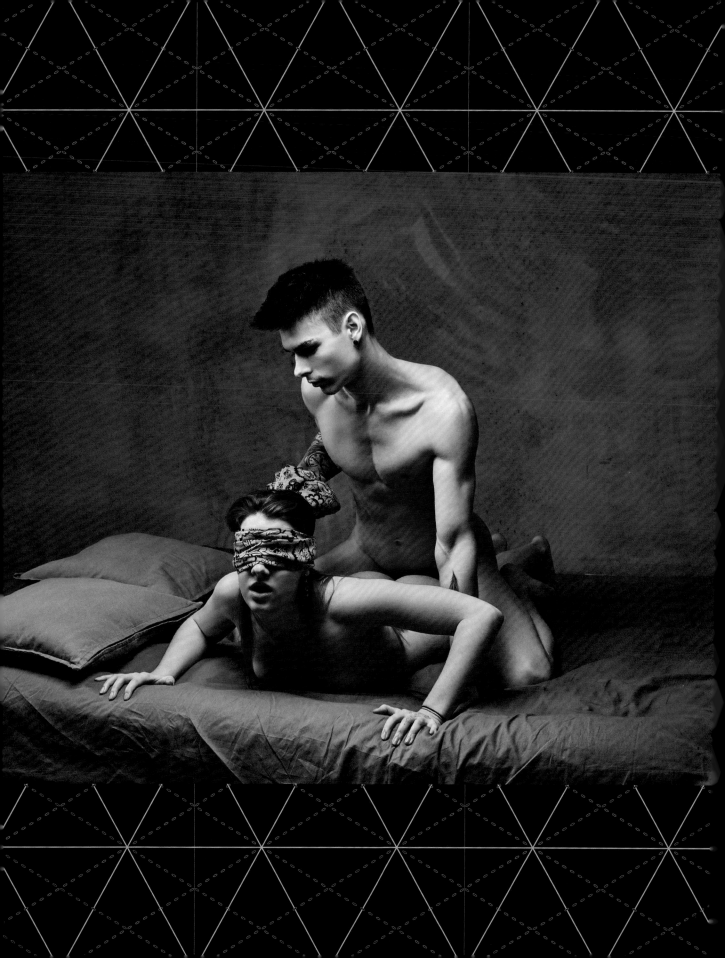

JOCKEY

The Jockey sex position is an old favorite for both rear-entry vaginal intercourse and anal sex. It's fun to do and comfortable for both partners. The position of her legs creates for a super-tight entrance either way, making it hotter for both him and her.

HOW TO DO IT

This is a fairly easy position to get into, and is exceptionally comfortable for the female partner. All she does is lie on her stomach with her legs together, and he does the rest. He will straddle her on his knees, with one knee on either side of her hips and one hand on either side of her shoulders. This is partly why it is called the Jockey sex position; it looks kind of like a jockey riding a racehorse!

WHERE TO DO IT

This is a great sex position for the bed, because it allows the female partner to be even more comfortable. But it can be done on the sofa, the floor, or anywhere else she has enough space to lie down.

PROPS YOU'LL NEED

She won't mind a pillow for her head, but it's not necessary. Optional blindfold and restraints are also a nice addition.

DIFFICULTY LEVEL ★☆☆☆☆

HER O-METER ★☆☆☆☆

While the Jockey is ultra-comfortable for her to get into and stay in, it really doesn't do much for her in the way of orgasms. Since she is face down, her clitoris is getting pretty much zero action, and unless she really digs rear entry vaginal intercourse or anal sex, this sex position is going to be something she does for him.

HIS O-METER ★★★★☆

He enjoys being in control here, and if he's a "butt guy," he's going to like this position even more. The tightness created by her legs being pressed together is a huge plus for him, too!

MAKE IT HOTTER . . .

This one is a lot of fun with a blindfold and restraints. Her hands can be restrained overhead or behind her back depending on her flexibility. If you tie them overhead, you can switch between Jockey and the next position, Missionary with a Twist, for some extra excitement.

MISSIONARY WITH A TWIST

This is a kinky variation of the basic Missionary sex position. The twist is that her hands (and/ or feet) are tied to the bed, or simply restrained in some way.

HOW TO DO IT

The traditional Missionary position is often known as "Man on Top." The male partner assumes the dominant position on top of the woman, who is lying on her back. Her legs are spread enough that her lover can thrust, but they're not raised up or resting on his shoulders. While she can thrust some, the primary work done is by the man. Because the Missionary is a very passive position for the female, it doesn't take much for the man to totally dominate her mentally and physically. The dominant sensation is increased even more when her hands and/or feet are restrained!

WHERE TO DO IT

The bed is best for this one.

PROPS YOU'LL NEED

Use soft ropes or silk ties for securing her to the bed.

DIFFICULTY LEVEL ★☆☆☆☆

HER O-METER ★★★★☆

Basic Missionary can be "boring" to say the least, but this "twist" really makes it hotter!

HIS O-METER ★★★★★

If he is a dominant man, he will love this. More timid men may feel overwhelmed by this one.

MAKE IT HOTTER . . .

Purchase an Under-the-Bed Restraint System to easily secure your lover whenever the desire strikes.

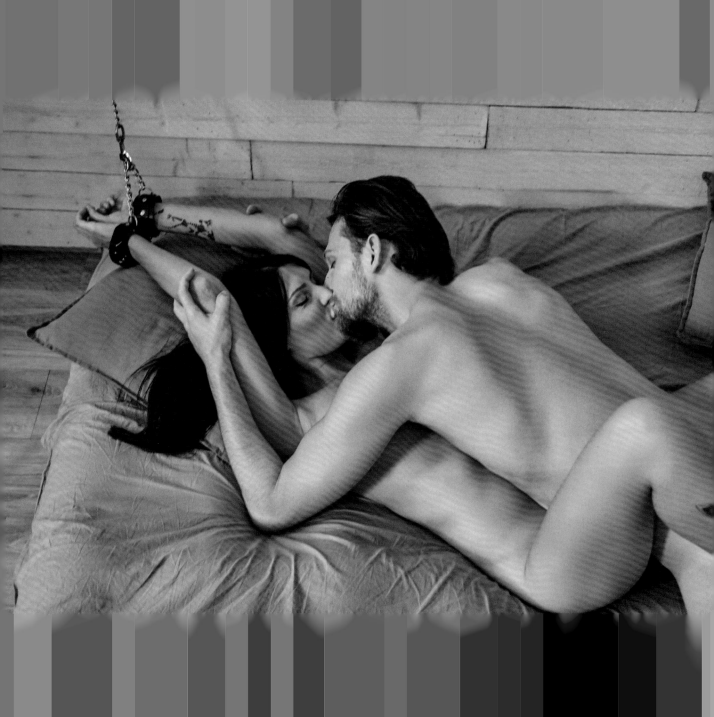

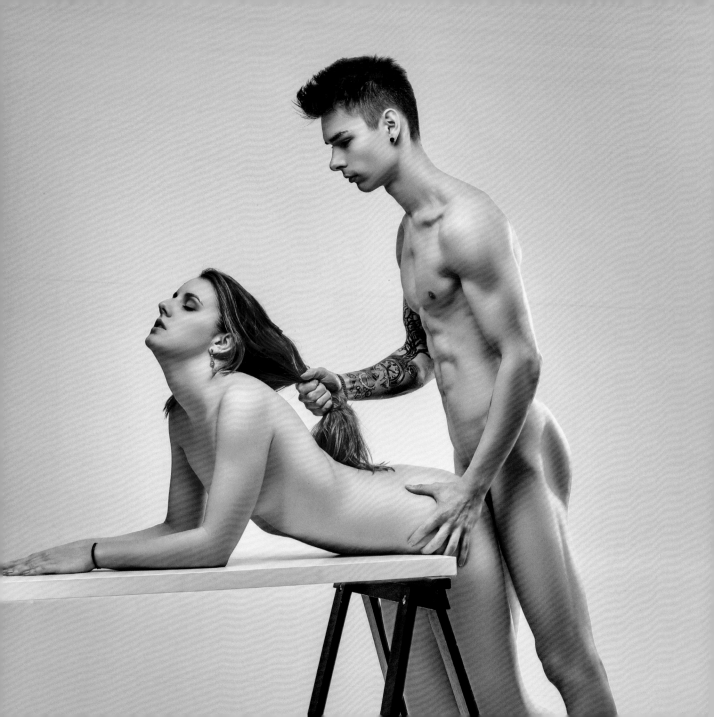

OVER THE DESK

The Over-the-Desk position is a kinky variation of Standing Doggy (see page 176). In this variation, the female partner is bent over a desk or table, and held down to introduce some light bondage into the position.

HOW TO DO IT

The female partner stands facing away from her partner and lays flat on the desk, table, or other raised surface. He enters her from behind while standing. It's very simple, but elicits exceptionally deep penetration and intense sensations for both partners.

WHERE TO DO IT

Do this one anywhere you can find a flat surface for her to lay over. Tables, desks, cars, or countertops are great options.

PROPS YOU'LL NEED

In addition to the flat surface, blindfolds, cuffs, or silk ties can increase the pleasure.

DIFFICULTY LEVEL ★☆☆☆☆

HER O-METER ★★★★☆

Women who enjoy being controlled, really deep penetration, and A-spot stimulation will get a lot out of the Over-the-Desk sex position. Women who are more timid or prefer lots of clitoral stimulation during intercourse won't like this one as much.

HIS O-METER ★★★★★

He loves to control her, and he loves the Standing-Doggy sex position just as much, if not more. He loves seeing her bent over just for him, and he loves grabbing her hips and thrusting deeply into her. He's in total control here, and the angle of penetration easily allows for him to insert his entire penis from tip to base. This is a must-try sex position for him!

MAKE IT HOTTER...

Try this one over the hood of the car (make sure it's cool to the touch), or bed of your truck. If you want to feel the thrill of public exposure without actually being exposed, you can do this while the car is in the garage. It's still incredibly hot!

DESK DOMINATION

While you have her laid out on your desk for Over The Desk, flip her over for a little Desk Domination.

HOW TO DO IT

The female partner lays flat on the desk on her back with her legs in the air like in Deep Victory, or wrapped around her partners back like Meet 'n' Greet. He can use her hips or the desk to help control the thrusting.

WHERE TO DO IT

Do this one anywhere you can find a flat surface for her to lay over. Tables, desks, cars, or countertops are great options. The trick is to find a surface that is at just the right height for easy thrusting. He will want to avoid reaching or bending down too far to avoid cramps.

PROPS YOU'LL NEED

In addition to the flat surface, blindfolds, cuffs, or silk ties can increase the pleasure.

DIFFICULTY LEVEL ★☆☆☆☆

HER O-METER ★★★★☆

The excitement from this position comes from the fact that he's in control. If she can truly let go and let him take charge, the intensity of this position is increased. Of course, she can always add in some clitoral stimulation and toys to help things along.

HIS O-METER ★★★★★

This is another great position for him because he is controlling the thrusting and movement. He has the added benefit of a standing position and a desk to hold on to for support.

MAKE IT HOTTER . . .

Tie her hands overhead to the underside of the desk, and tease her orally just to the point of orgasm before entering her, and then make her wait just a minute or so before that first powerful thrust. She may just explode with orgasm on that first thrust.

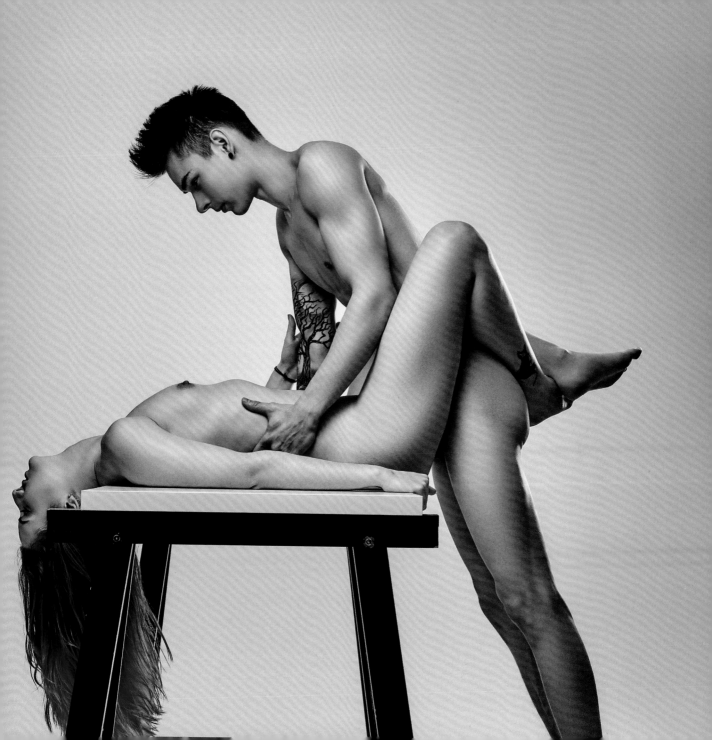

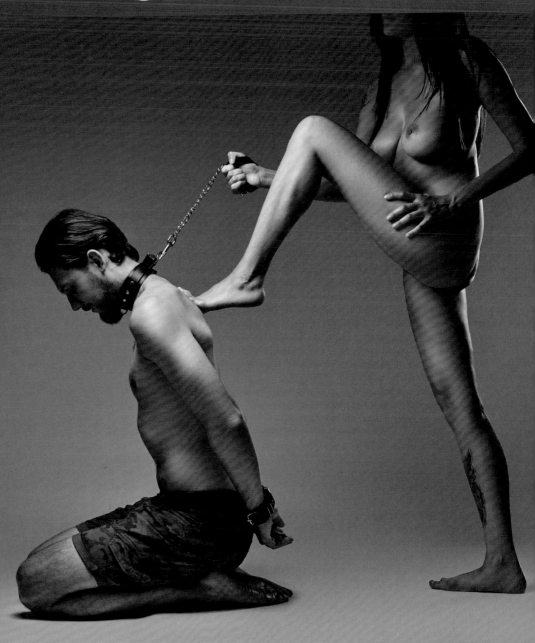

SEXY CHALLENGE:

CHAIN OF COMMAND

Bondage is a subject that is fascinating and scary for many couples. We are all a little curious about the subject, but we often fail to understand that you don't have to jump into it full-blown. There are several different, yet simple, things to help you introduce bondage into your relationship that are not as threatening as many of the things we see on television or the internet. Did you know that something as simple as a blindfold can be considered bondage? Many consider bondage to be whips and chains and floggers, oh my, but the simple fact is that anything that takes away some form of control of one person can be considered bondage. In the case of the blindfold, you are taking away the power of the person to see. Thus, they don't know when or where their lover is going to touch them next, or with what they are going to touch them. If you have a blindfold, welcome to the world of bondage.

Obviously, the blindfold is on the very vanilla end of the bondage chart. You can branch out into cock rings, harnesses, silk ropes, floggers, ball gags, spreader bars, bondage clothing, and even bondage furniture. The list of bondage accessories is long and quite interesting. However, if you are new to this arena, I suggest you take it slowly. That is what the Sexy Challenge Chain of Command is all about: allowing you to wade into the pool of bondage without being thrown into the deep end. The Chain of Command is designed for partners to experiment, and gradually see where their own comfort level stops. So, the first thing you need to do is purchase links of actual chain. You can get chain at your local hardware store, and they will most likely cost you only a few bucks. Just make sure you get the cheapest chain you can get; the quality is not important, as we are not going to be using the chain in actual bondage situations. I had you scared a little, didn't I?

Once you have picked out your chain, cut the chain so that you have two sections that have ten links each. There will be one section of chain for each partner for this challenge. You can be creative with your chain if you like, and paint it so that you can tell them apart if you wish. Now, each partner takes their chain and individually goes to a location in the house where they have a computer with internet access. In their own privacy, each partner now will do some research on bondage. They each need to find ten things that they are willing to try, and then rank them in order from one to ten, with ten being the most intense thing you think you would be willing to try. Now, these can be actual items, such as those mentioned above, or they can be actions, such as starting out by having your partner slap your ass with their bare hand. Once you have your ten items listed in order, you need to realize that each item will correspond with a link on your chain! Now you can meet back up with your partner and share lists.

Each partner will go over the other partner's list and pass no judgement. The important part here is to have open communication. Remember, just because your partner might want to be tied up and suspended from the ceiling, doesn't mean you have to do it. Now, as you look down your lists, you need to start collecting any items that you might need to start this journey. If you're a little nervous to go to a store and purchase these items, don't worry; that is why the internet was invented.

Once you have the items you need, you will be ready to begin the Ten-Day Chain-of-Command Sexy Challenge. Next, pick out ten days on the calendar for your experimentation to begin. On the first day, start with your number-one desire, and start working your way down the list each consecutive day.

Since this is new to you, then you have to understand that at any point your partner can tell you to stop, or decide they are uncomfortable with their choice, and if that is the case, you have to respect that and stop. When that happens, it doesn't mean the fun has to stop; you can at that point go back to your normal, sexually-exciting fun. Remember, there is no shame here; we are experimenting with the Chain of Command to see how we react to it and to see what kind of bondage we are OK with in our relationship.

Continue this process for the ten-day cycle. Each day you complete an activity and think you wouldn't mind doing that again, cut a link of your chain off. Do the same for your partner's chain for these ten days. At the end of the ten days, compare your chains to see how many links are remaining. If you have no links left, congrats—you are a bondage freak, and you might want to do this challenge again to experience more. If you only have one to three links left, it is pretty obvious that you are OK with bondage being part of your sexual relationship. If you have four-to-six links remaining, bondage is something that you will enjoy, but not all the time; maybe for special occasions or just on those nights you are really feeling randy. Now, if you have seven-to-nine links remaining, you might stay more into the shallow end of the bondage pool, and stick with the blindfolds and mild restraints.

If you still have ten links left, it is obvious you didn't find any bondage items that excited you this time. Now, that doesn't mean you are never to try again; it just means at this point and time, and with what you picked, you didn't enjoy it. If, as a couple, you have very different chain links at the end of the Sexy Challenge Chain of Command, don't think you have to break up and find someone different. Understand it is OK to like different things. Maybe your partner loves the feel of a cock ring that isn't going to hurt you while you are making love; maybe your partner loves to be tied up, and if they do, you can tie them up and give them pleasure, which can be a huge turn on for you, even though you don't like being tied up. The big point with the Sexy

Challenge Chain of Command is carving out the items that work well in your unique relationship; it doesn't matter what anyone else thinks or does—this is about you and your partner, and what kinky things you do together is your business.

Chapter 13: Advanced Topics and Positions for the Truly Adventurous

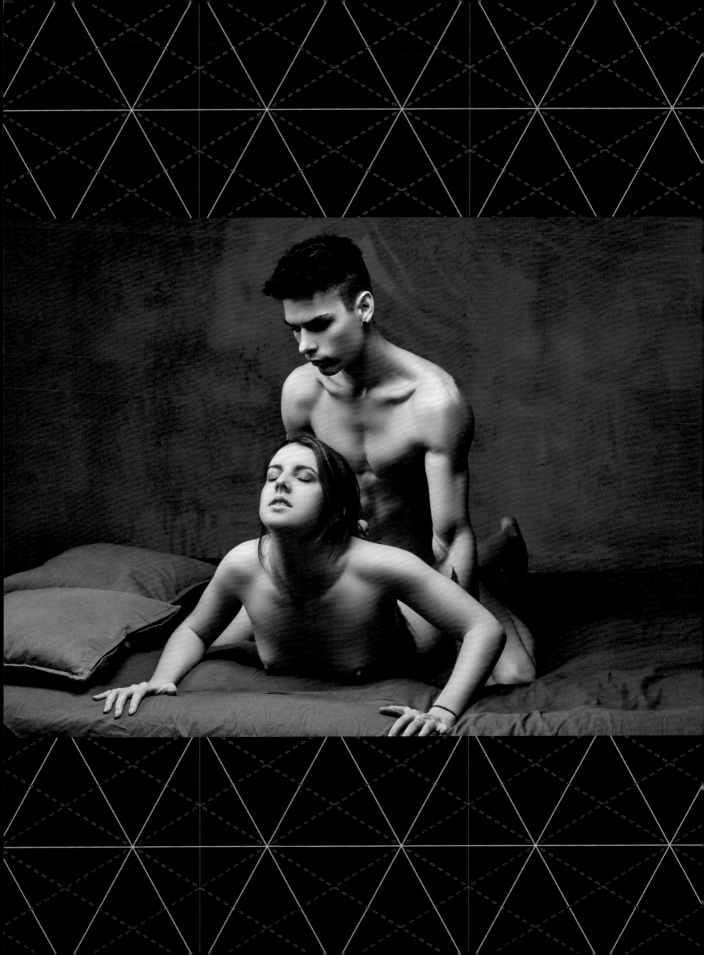

Anal Sex

Anal sex is one of those topics that's guaranteed to cause a debate; some people love it and some people hate it. I personally believe everyone should try it at least twice before taking a stance. It feels good, while at the same time triggering all of those "naughty" thrills that keep your sex life interesting. An added bonus is that with the help of toys, both male and female partners can enjoy receiving anal sex.

HOW TO DO IT

Anal sex can be performed in just about any position where you can have vaginal sex, but to get started, I recommend either Basic Rear Entry or Doggy Style. If the receiving partner wants a little more control of the thrusting and penetration, then Cowgirl works well too.

Hygiene is critical for everyone to feel comfortable with anal sex. Take a shower and wash thoroughly before getting started. I also recommend an anal douche to flush out your anus if you want to be extra clean.

The reason that many people do not like anal sex is because it can hurt if you move too fast and don't use enough lube. Take your time, and use lots and lots of lube or coconut oil. Start with your fingers or a small anal toy to get used to the sensations. Once you start to relax, only then move on to larger toys or penis. Again, take it slow and be very gentle. It can feel a little intense at first, but as things relax back there, you can pick up the pace.

WHERE TO DO IT

The bed is a great place to start, but the floor or bending over a table or chair works equally well.

PROPS YOU'LL NEED

Different sizes of toys and a good lube. Oil and silicon-based lubes work really well, but a good water-based lube is good too.

DIFFICULTY LEVEL ★★☆☆☆

HER O-METER ★★★☆☆

If she is willing to relax and let go of her inhibitions, anal sex can be very pleasurable and highly orgasmic. Anal sex allows easy access for clitoral stimulation, as well as extra vaginal stimulation for maximum pleasure.

HIS O-METER ★★★☆☆

Most men really enjoy giving anal sex. Maybe it's the excitement of doing something taboo, or the extreme physical pleasure, but I've yet to meet a man who's tried anal sex who doesn't absolutely love it.

Receiving anal sex can be a tough topic, especially for heterosexual men, but like I said above, try it twice before you take a stand. We'll go into this more in the section on Pegging.

MAKE IT HOTTER . . .

Anal sex truly opens up the possibilities! Adding clitoral stimulation, and additional vaginal penetration from a toy or another penis, can really rock her world.

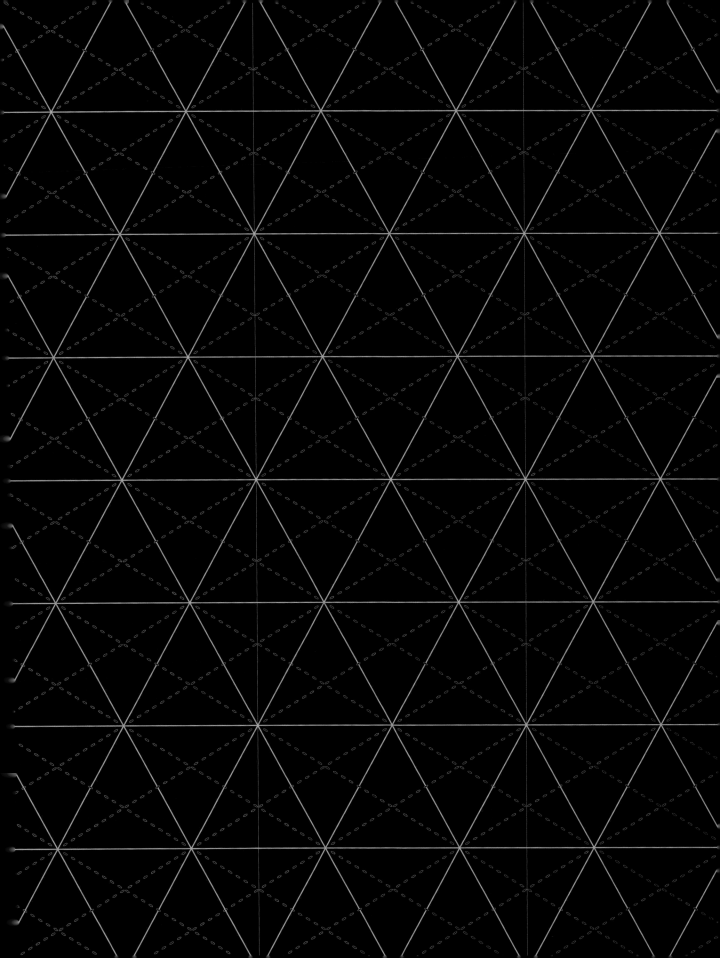

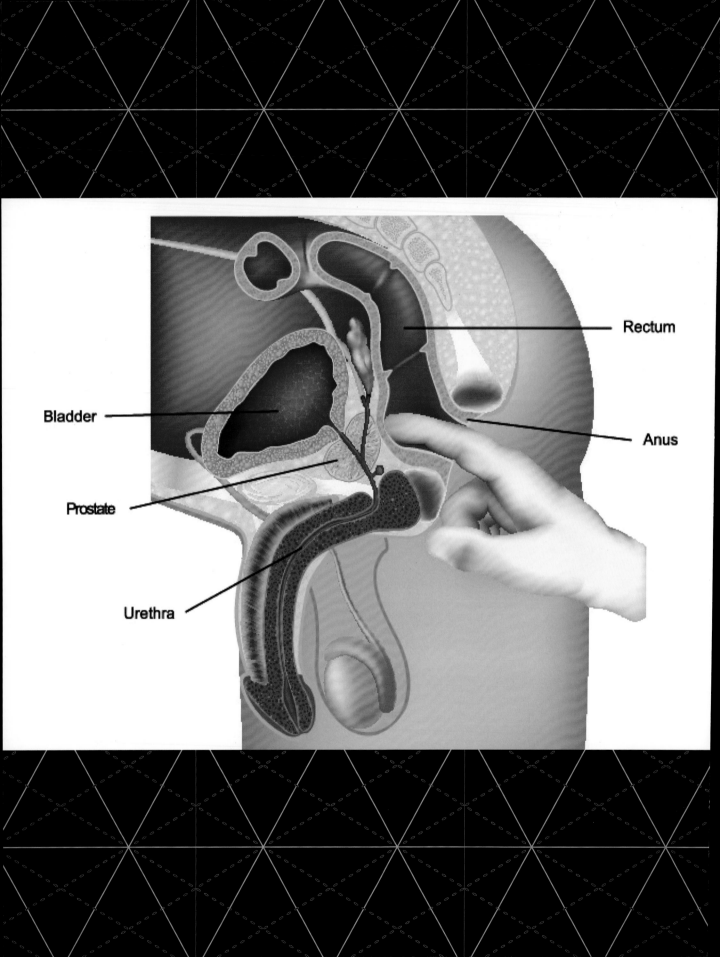

Rectum

Anus

Bladder

Prostate

Urethra

PROSTATE MILKING

Prostate milking is a fairly simply process that involves applying light-to-moderate pressure to the prostate gland. The prostate gland is most easily accessed through the anus. It's just inside the anus, about two knuckles into the rectum. It sits on the front side of the body. The goal here is to find and slowly massage the prostate gland. Every man is different and it will take some practice to find just the right spot and pressure for maximum pleasure.

HOW TO DO IT

To access your prostate gland yourself, simply lay in bed on your side, and pull the knee of your upper leg toward your chest. Then, you can more easily insert your finger or favorite anal toy. Using plenty of lube makes things flow more smoothly. I personally like a good silicon-based lube for anal play.

The prostate can also be massaged from the outside, though the intensity may not be as strong.

An external prostate massage can be achieved by applying direct pressure to the perineum, that section of skin between the anus and scrotum. You can do this with your fingertips or a toy. Make sure to use a good lube or natural oil and start with light pressure. As above, contract and relax your muscles as you massage this area. Pay attention to the sensations and let your body guide you.

WHERE TO DO IT

When you're just getting started, the best place to learn prostate massage is in your bed or on the sofa, at home where you can be completely relaxed and comfortable.

PROPS YOU'LL NEED

A good silicon lube, an anal toy that is about three-to-four inches long with a bulbous end.

DIFFICULTY LEVEL ★☆☆☆☆

It will take a bit of practice, but once you figure this out, it's not difficult.

HER O-METER ★☆☆☆☆

This one's all for him, so her pleasure will come from experiencing his pleasure with him.

HIS O-METER ★★★★★

A prostate orgasm can be incredibly pleasurable for him.

MAKE IT HOTTER...

Insert an anal toy to massage his prostate while he is inside of her. Once you're comfortable, try this with some sitting positions like Laptop for extra intensity.

HERE'S SOME TIPS TO GET STARTED WITH PROSTATE MILKING:

Apply a generous amount of lube to your anus and the toy or fingers.

Gently ease the toy into your anus. Take your time and go slow. Most anal toys are larger at the end, so once you get past the initial insertion, it gets way more comfortable! You can also use your fingers to get the anus to relax a bit before trying to insert the toy.

Contract and release your groin muscles around the toy as if you're trying to stop and start the flow of urine. This will draw the toy in and out, massaging your prostate. Breathing with the rhythm of your contractions can really help with the flow of energy into and out of your body.

Once you find the right rhythm and strength of contractions, you will eventually achieve the end goal of an incredible orgasm. It may not happen the first time, but keep practicing and you will be rewarded.

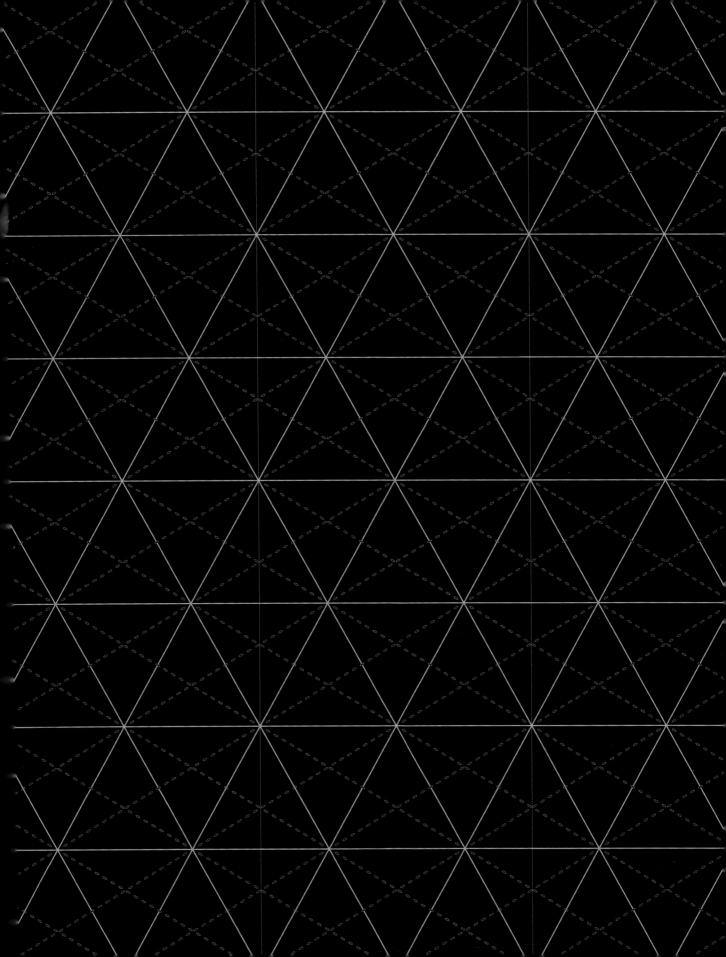

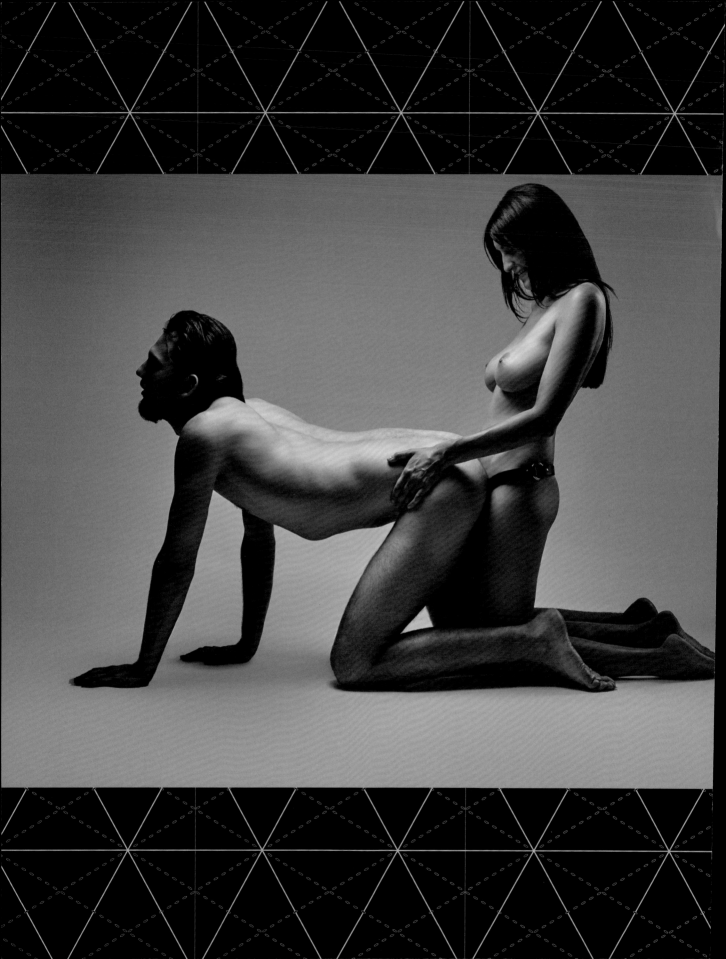

PEGGING

Pegging is quite simply when a woman penetrates a man in the anus with a strap-on dildo. The idea can be uncomfortable for some straight men because anal sex is often considered a homosexual sex act. This is just not true. In this scenario, it is just straight sex between a man and a woman.

Anal sex, no matter what your gender, is enjoyable if performed correctly. There are so many nerve endings and pleasure points in and around the anus that it can amazing! It may even feel better for a man to receive anal sex because the prostate gland resides inside the male anus. A man can achieve orgasm purely by stimulating the prostate gland without any penis contact at all.

HOW TO DO IT

Pegging can be performed in just about any position, but to get started, I recommend Doggy Style or Standing Doggy Style because, let's face it, women are not as experienced when it comes to thrusting, so keep it simple at first.

Hygiene is critical for everyone to feel comfortable with any sort of anal play. Take a shower and wash thoroughly before getting started. I also recommend an anal douche to flush out your anus, if you want to be extra clean.

Once again, take your time, and use lots and lots of lube or coconut oil. Start with your fingers or a small anal toy to get used to the sensations. Once you start to relax, only then move on to larger toys or penis. Again, take it slow and be very gentle. It can feel a little intense at first, but as things relax back there, you can pick up the pace.

WHERE TO DO IT

On the bed, or bent over a table or chair.

PROPS YOU'LL NEED

A good strap-on dildo and harness are required for basic pegging. Different sizes of toys and a good lube are as well. Oil and silicon-based lubes work really well, but a good water-based lube is good, too.

DIFFICULTY LEVEL ★★☆☆☆

HER O-METER ★★☆☆☆

There's not going to be much actual orgasmic pleasure for her, but it can still be highly arousing and fun. Some women can orgasm just from the pressure and friction of the harness, but not all can. A bullet vibrator can also be added to the inside of the harness to add pleasure for her.

HIS O-METER ★★★★☆

If he can let go of his inhibitions around getting penetrated in the ass by a woman, pegging can be highly orgasmic for a man. Many men can orgasm just from having the prostate gland stimulated. It's a lot like the G-spot for a woman.

MAKE IT HOTTER . . .

Try a double-ended dildo so that you can both experience penetration at the same time! You'll have to change up the position to something like the Crab or Lotus, but the sensations are incredible!

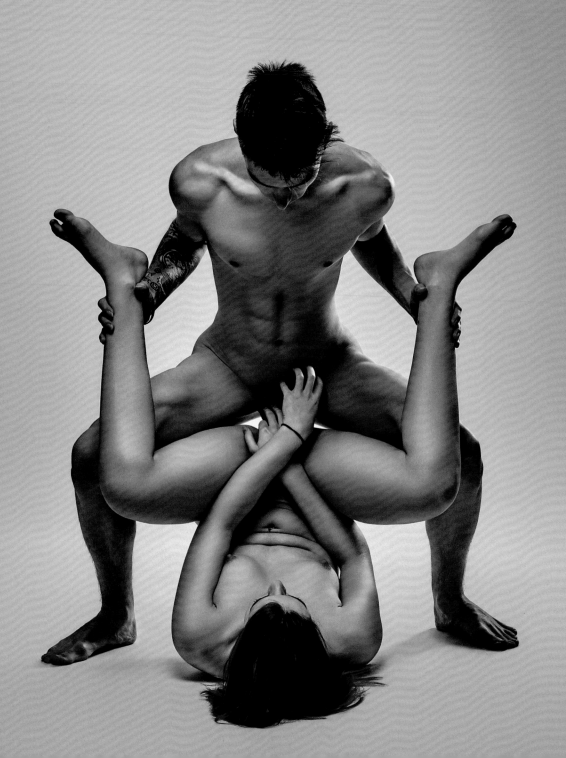

BUTTER CHURNER

The Butter-Churner is an advanced sex position, in which the woman lies on her back with her legs raised above and behind her head. The man then squats and penetrates her from above. The thrusting motion in this position is similar to making butter in an old-fashioned butter churner, which is how this position gets its name.

HOW TO DO IT

The woman lies on her back with her legs raised and folded over so that her ankles are on either side of her head. He squats and takes his penis in and out of her vagina.

WHERE TO DO IT

A stable surface like the floor is best for this position.

PROPS YOU'LL NEED

A pillow or cushion to go under her shoulder and head will make this a lot more bearable for her.

DIFFICULTY LEVEL ★★★★★

The Butter Churner is a physically demanding position for both partners. It requires significant neck and shoulder flexibility from her, and leg strength and balance from him.

HER O-METER ★★★★☆

The increased blood flow to her head can greatly increase her ecstasy level. It's a similar feeling to breath control or a hand around your throat. However, he needs to be very cautious in this position to avoid thrusting too hard or putting too much pressure on her neck.

HIS O-METER ★★☆☆☆

He's not likely to orgasm in the position. It's more about the bragging rights that he did it.

MAKE IT HOTTER . . .

Do this in front of a full-length mirror,--------- or dribble chocolate syrup or honey into her mouth.

SNOW ANGEL

Ready to make your own snow angel? You're going to love this challenging sex position.

HOW TO DO IT

There are two options to do the Snow Angel. For the first option, she lies on her back in a spread-eagle position, then he does the same thing on top of her, only facing in the opposite direction toward her feet. The modification allows both partners to bend their knees a little more. This also allows her to tilt her hips upward to allow him to more easily penetrate her. Once in position, the movement is more of a rocking motion than a traditional thrusting motion.

WHERE TO DO IT

On the bed or floor is best for this position.

PROPS YOU'LL NEED

If you're doing the modified version of the snow angel, a pillow or cushion under her hips will help with the angle of insertion.

DIFFICULTY LEVEL ★★★★☆

This is a very challenging position. His penis needs to be flexible and on the longer side for this position to work.

HER O-METER ★★★☆☆

This position allows her to position herself in such a way that his penis or scrotum rubs her clitoris during the motion, making it possible to achieve a strong orgasm.

HIS O-METER ★★☆☆☆

Because of the angle of insertion, this will not be his favorite position unless he enjoys a good prostate massage.

MAKE IT HOTTER . . .

This is the perfect position to insert a finger or toy into his anus and to give him a wonderful prostate massage.

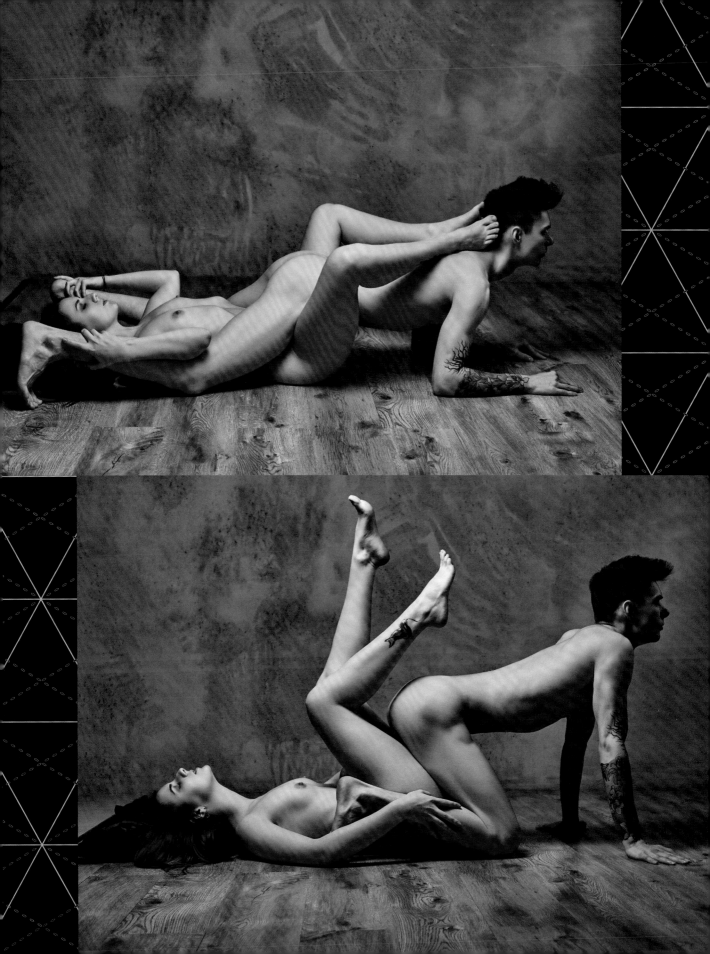

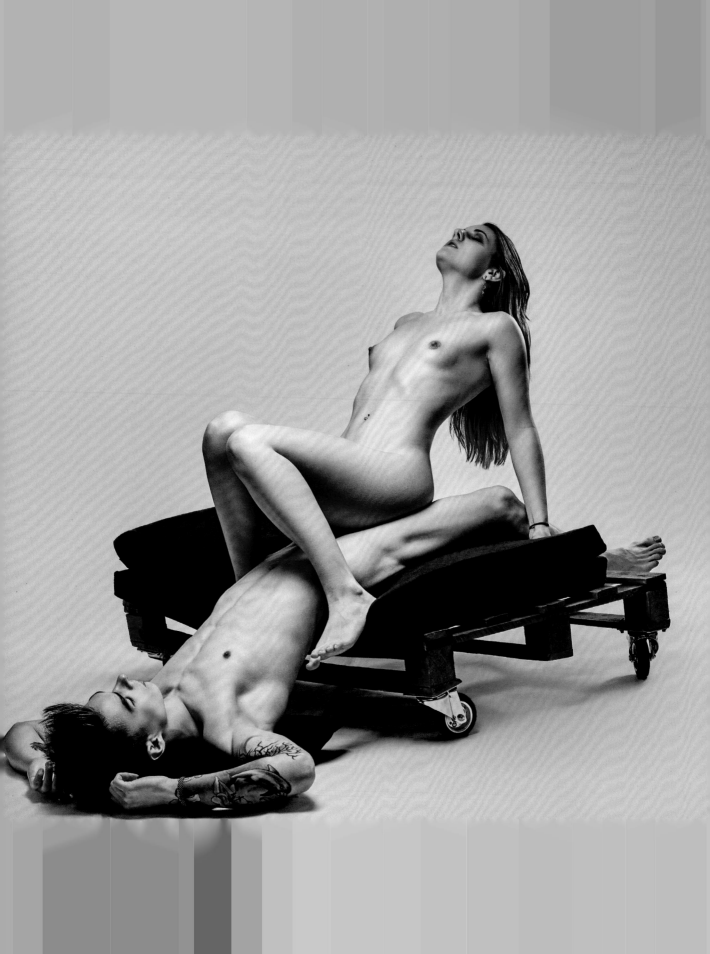

WATERFALL

While there are many variations of this position, I prefer the woman-on-top variation. It's a very orgasmic position for both partners because she gets to control the depth and angle of penetration, and he gets the extra rush of blood to his head. Both of these combine for a very climactic ending.

HOW TO DO IT

To get into this position, the male partner lies on his back, with his head and torso off the edge of the bed. His shoulders can rest on the ground but they don't have to. She straddles him with her legs in front similar to the Crab sex position (page 50) and slides forward so that her weight is primarily on her feet.

WHERE TO DO IT

A low bed, ottoman, or sofa work best for this position.

PROPS YOU'LL NEED

A pillow to go under his shoulders for comfort. You can also work up to this position by starting out on two-to-three sofa cushions and gradually increasing the height as you get more comfortable with the position.

DIFFICULTY LEVEL ★★★★★

HER O-METER ★★★★☆

This position allows her to be in control of depth and angle penetration. She is in control of her orgasm. Once she orgasms, she can then focus on what he needs and wants to make the position more pleasurable for him.

HIS O-METER ★★★★☆

The position allows for a great view and the blood rush to his head enhances the sensation and orgasm.

MAKE IT HOTTER...

He already has an amazing view, but she can make it even better by caressing her own body and clitoris. The more she gets into it, the more he will enjoy it.

SHOULDER STAND

The shoulder stand is the man-on-top variation of the Waterfall. While traditionally a stranding position, it can be done from a seated or kneeling position to make it easier for both partners.

HOW TO DO IT

If you've ever seen a shoulder stand in yoga, then you have a pretty good understanding of this position. He stands on his knees at her feet. She gets into a shoulder stand, and rests her feet on his shoulders or chest. He supports her hips to provide stability and control thrusting. She should arch her back to make penetration more achievable.

WHERE TO DO IT

The floor is best for this position because a solid surface is critical to get into and maintain this position.

PROPS YOU'LL NEED

A pillow can be placed under her shoulders for comfort. A yoga ball can help her to stay in this position and maintain a good arch in her back. It will also take some of the strain off her back. A good modification for this position is for him to sit on his knees on the sofa or ottoman (or even some sofa cushions), and have her sit on his lap and then lean back until her shoulders are on the floor.

DIFFICULTY LEVEL ★★★★★

HER O-METER ★★★★☆

This position is a great angle for G-spot stimulation, so if she's in good enough shape to hold the position and still relax enough to have an orgasm, those orgasms can be quite powerful.

HIS O-METER ★★★★☆

He is control of thrusting depth, angle, and speed, so if she can maintain the position long enough, he will love this position!

MAKE IT HOTTER . . .

A butt plug is a great addition here for her (or him). She can also squeeze or tickle his nipples with her toes.

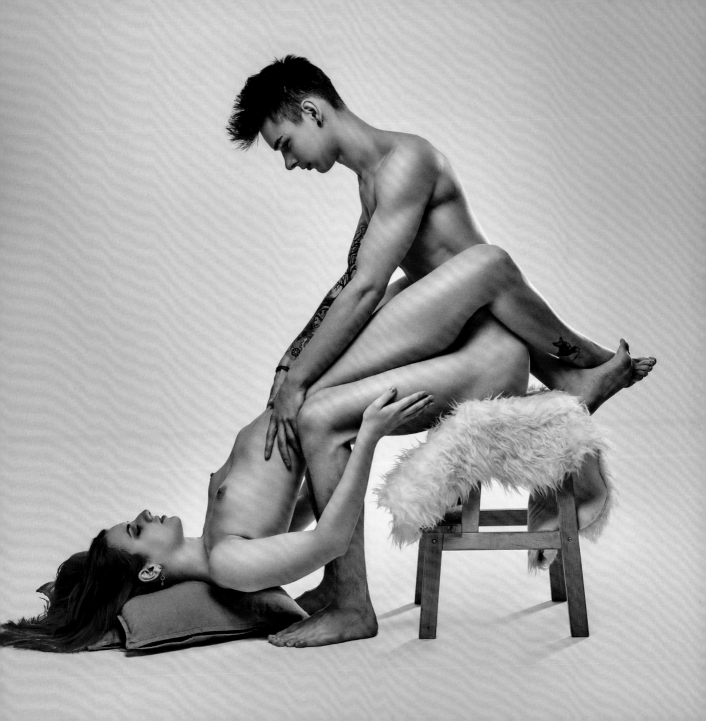

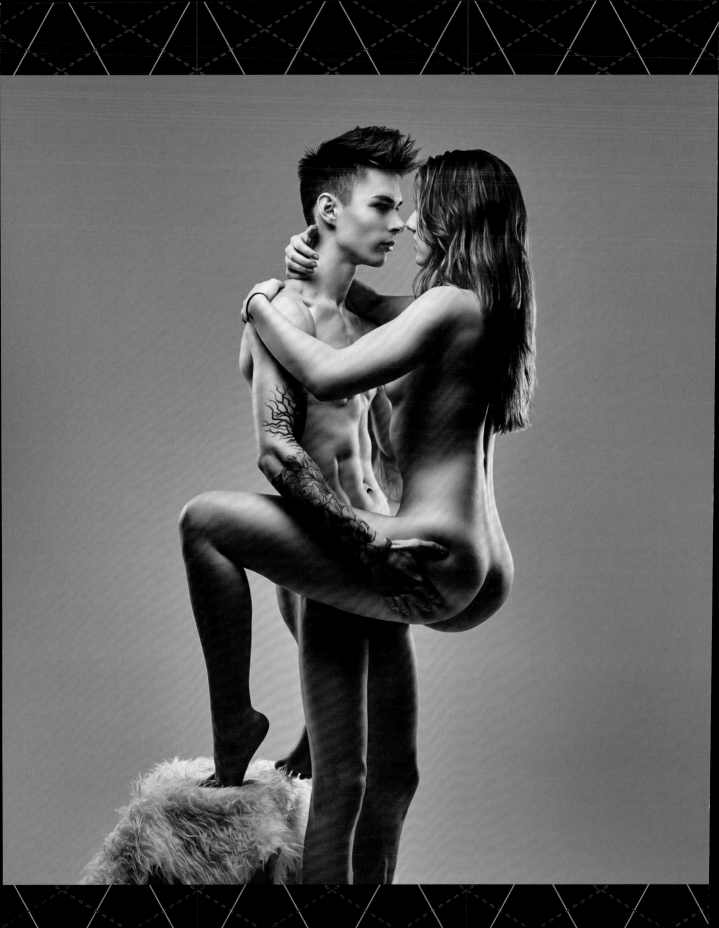

THE HANGING GARDEN

The man takes full control with the Hanging-Garden sex position. This position is physically demanding for him but well worth it because it's one of the all-time sexiest standing positions!

HOW TO DO IT

He picks her up and holds her in position while she wraps her legs around his waist and helps support her weight by wrapping her hands or arms around his neck.

WHERE TO DO IT

This is a great position for small spaces where you do not have room to lie or sit down like a closet to shower. Please be very careful in the shower as this position is very challenging both in strength and balance.

PROPS YOU'LL NEED

Leaning her against the wall or other stable surface like a countertop can help make this position more stable. This position works best when he is much stronger and larger than she is because it requires a lot of upper body strength to make this position really work well. The Laptop sex position is a good modification if this one simply is not possible.

DIFFICULTY LEVEL ★★★★★

HER O-METER ★★★★★

This position can be very orgasmic for her, especially if she is highly aroused before getting into this position.

HIS O-METER ★★★★★

His ability to orgasm in this position will be directly related to his strength and stamina. It's an incredibly sexy position and he's in control, but if he tires out, it just won't happen for him.

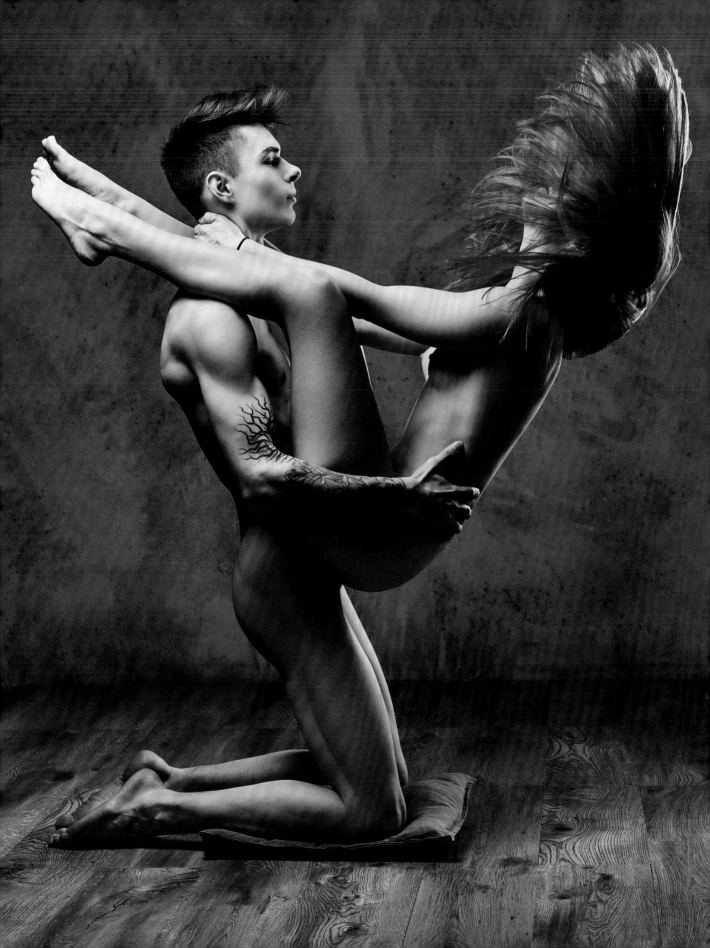

MAKE IT HOTTER . . .

Feeling super ambitious? Take this to the next level by getting down on your knees. It will provide a whole new angle of thrusting and provide an amazing glutei workout!

WHEELBARROW

The Wheelbarrow is definitely a favorite for guys who enjoy exotic sex positions, even though it might not be one of her favorites. With him in total control, she's at his mercy! It's an excellent position for guys who really like a "butt view."

HOW TO DO IT

The male partner stands normally, with his feet about shoulder width apart. The female partner will get on all fours, à la Doggy Style, and back up to him until she's close enough that he can bend down and pick her up from the waist. From there, he will position her hips in line with his, entering her from "behind." This requires a bit of strength on his part, but it shouldn't be too difficult. She will spread her legs out, allowing him to get a good grip on her hips and thighs to allow for thrusting. Her hands are still positioned on the floor, supporting the majority of her weight.

WHERE TO DO IT

Try this one a room with plenty of space and no furniture in the way. The Wheelbarrow sex position definitely requires one thing, and that's space!

PROPS YOU'LL NEED

She might want a towel, soft blanket, or rug to put under her hands to prevent rug burn or palm irritation. A sex swing is a terrific additional to make this position more approachable for most people.

DIFFICULTY LEVEL ★★★★☆

HER O-METER ★☆☆☆☆

There's not much in it for her as far as the Wheelbarrow goes. It's an awkward position for her to get into, and for her to stay in. The blood will rush to her head, making her a little dizzy, and she may not be able to keep it up for long. However, some women who enjoy exotic positions will certainly dig the novelty here.

HIS O-METER ★★★☆☆

He is in complete control of sex in this position, and he loves it! The view is great, he's comfortable standing up, and it's just all around a super-hot sex position for him, and assuming he has the physical fitness to truly enjoy the position, he'll really like it.

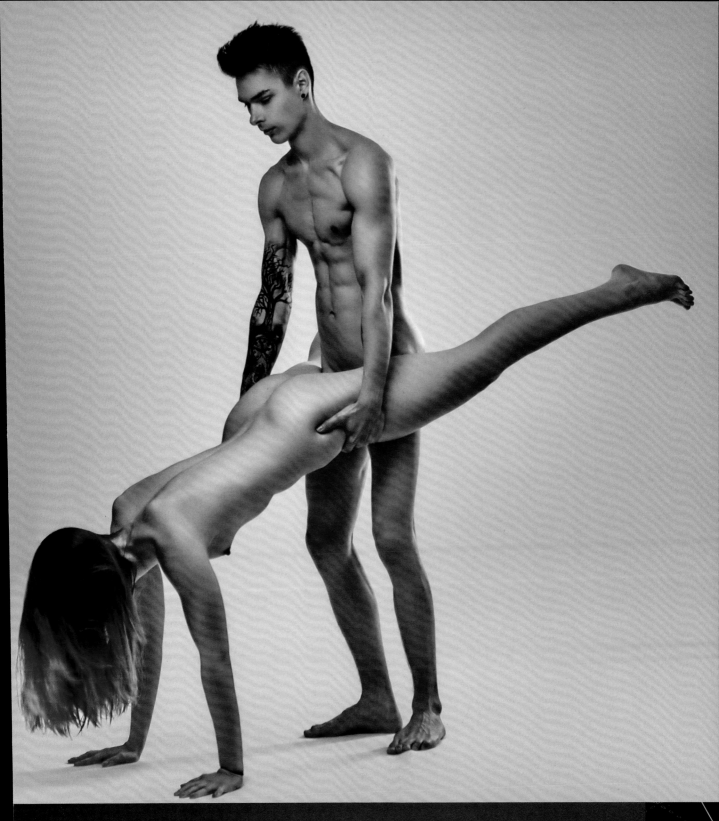

MAKE IT HOTTER . . .

This is a really fun position to do in a sex swing! It will give her some support and allow for more robust thrusting when both partners are not worried about falling over.

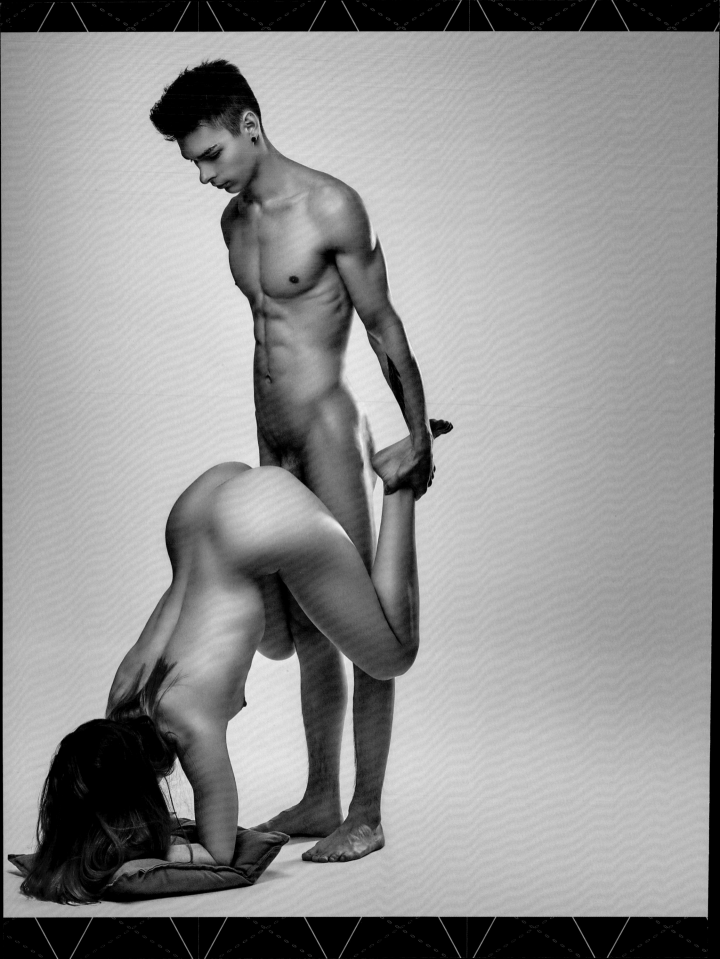

PLOW

Like the Wheelbarrow sex position? Then you may just love the Plow.

HOW TO DO IT

As with the Wheelbarrow sex position, the male partner stands normally, with his feet about shoulder width apart. The female partner will get on all fours, à la Doggy Style, and back up to him until she's close enough that he can bend down and pick her up from the feet. From there, he will position her hips in line with his, entering her from "behind." Instead of getting up on her hands, she will stay on her elbows this time. Because her weight is on her elbows and her knees are bent, she can actually help with the thrusting, or control it all together.

WHERE TO DO IT

Anywhere you can stand up and not worry about falling over onto furniture.

PROPS YOU'LL NEED

She might want a towel, soft blanket, or rug to put under her elbows to prevent rug burn or palm irritation.

DIFFICULTY LEVEL ★★★★☆

HER O-METER ★★☆☆☆

This is a very physically demanding position, so for most women, orgasms will be hard to achieve for those women who are not yoga masters and accustomed to having their weight inverted.

HIS O-METER ★★★★☆

Like the Wheelbarrow, his view is great, he's comfortable standing up, and it's just all around a super-hot sex position for him so long as he is fit enough to enjoy it.

MAKE IT HOTTER . . .

Once again, a sex swing is a terrific addition to make this position more approachable for most people, especially if there is a large height difference between the two partners.

BRIDGE

A guy will love the show a woman gives him when she bends over backwards in the Bridge sex position. It's a fairly difficult position to master, especially for women. However, longevity is not necessary in this position—it's a great one to try for a little while before you switch to something else.

HOW TO DO IT

The female partner will place her hands and feet on the floor while lying on her back and push herself up into a "bridge" position, with her back arched and stomach curved towards the ceiling. The male partner kneels, aligns himself with his partner, and gently guides her hips as he thrusts. In this sex position, the female partner can lose her balance quite easily, and only very flexible women will be able to comfortably have sex in this position. However, her arched back and exposed body give him a very nice view!

WHERE TO DO IT

The floor is excellent for this position.

PROPS YOU'LL NEED

Placing an ottoman or yoga ball under her back for support can help her stay in this position longer.

DIFFICULTY LEVEL ★★★★★

HER O-METER ★☆☆☆☆

This can be an extremely uncomfortable sex position for a woman to get into, even if she is flexible. She may only be able to keep it up for a few minutes at a time, which is completely normal. Ladies, if you find this sex position just doesn't do it for you, don't be surprised. It's difficult! Even if you do achieve this position and can keep it up for some time, the angle of penetration doesn't provide for good clitoral or G-spot stimulation. This one's more of a novelty for your guy.

HIS O-METER ★★★★☆

He will love how exotic this sex position is. It's almost as if his partner is splayed out just for his viewing enjoyment, and in a way, she is! Since she gets very little out of this sex position, it's pretty much all for him.

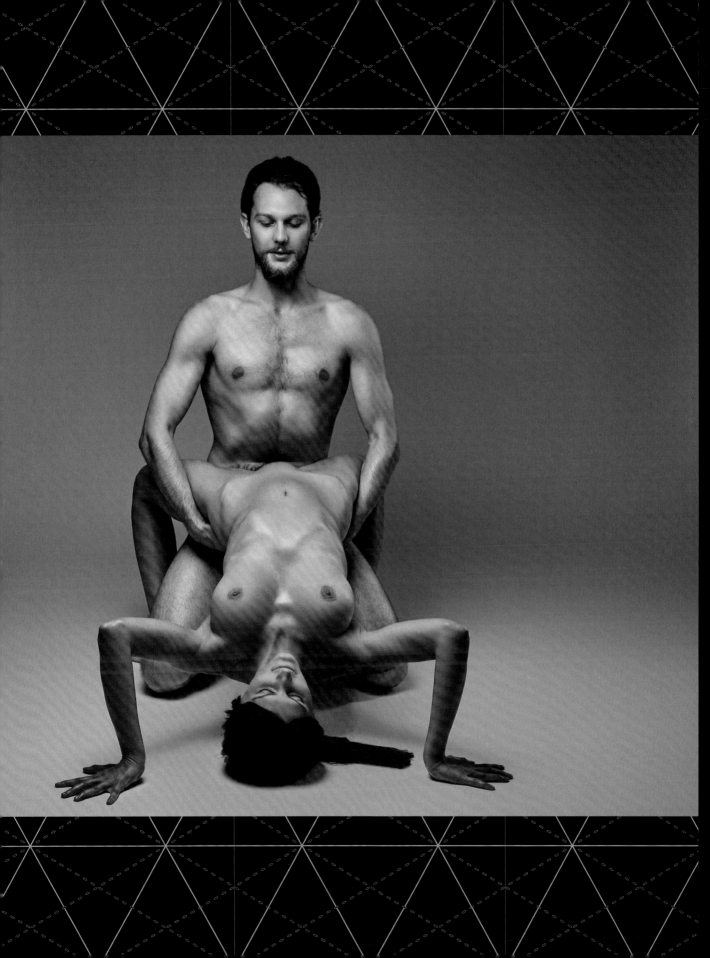

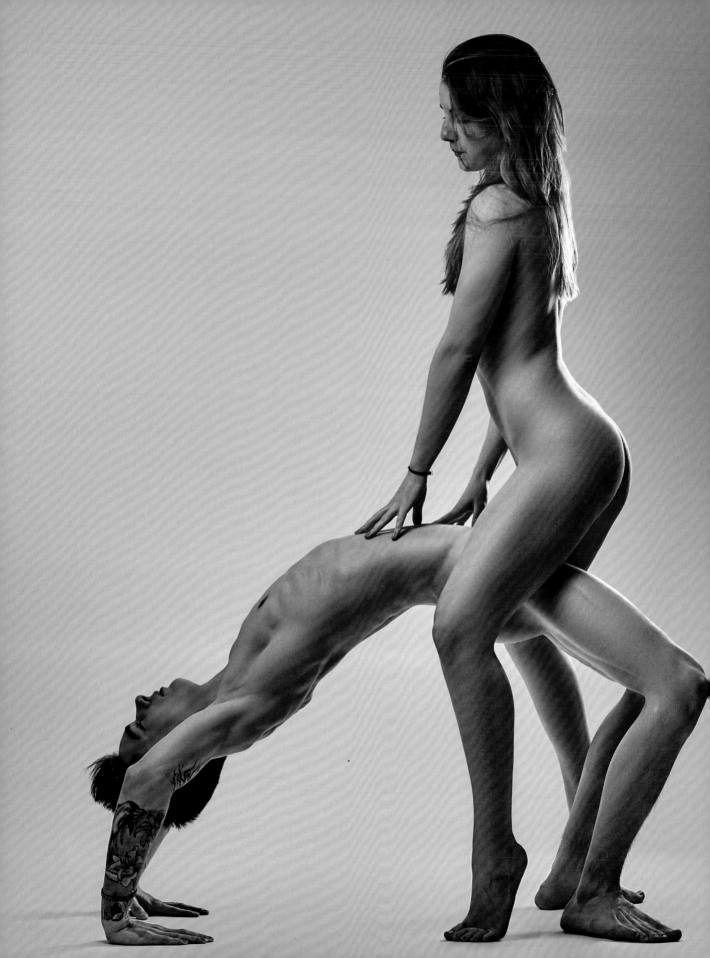

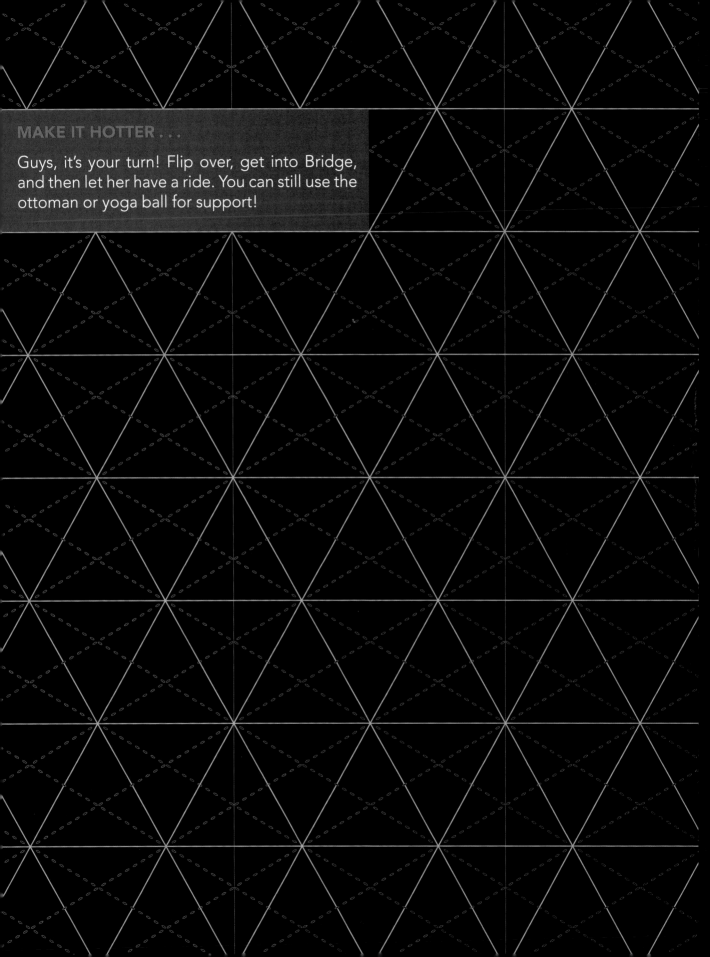

MAKE IT HOTTER . . .

Guys, it's your turn! Flip over, get into Bridge, and then let her have a ride. You can still use the ottoman or yoga ball for support!

TEN SEX TOYS EVERY COUPLE SHOULD OWN

328 ten sex toys every couple should own

Jennifer's List

1. LELO SORAYA

The Lelo Soraya is the best clitoral and G-spot vibrator on the market, both in terms of function and quality of materials. If you can have only one sex toy, this is the one. I've tried hundreds of toys over the years, and this is one that I go back to again and again.

www.lelo.com/soraya

2. LELO SONA

The Lelo Sona is one of the most popular new style of vibrators on the market today. Instead of mechanical vibrations, it uses sonic waves and pulses to create intense stimulation. As an added bonus, it's completely waterproof!

www.lelo.com/sona

3. JIMMYJANE FORM 2

The Form 2 is my hands-down favorite clitoral vibrator! This may sound odd, but to me, it looks like a giant tooth, only way more sexy! It has two nubs that each vibrate with several programmable patterns, so that you can find the perfect placement and sensation. And it's also completely waterproof!

www.jimmyjane.com/form-2-rechargeable-vibrator

4. PINKCHERRY DOUBLE G GLASS DILDO STUNNER

Everyone should have at least one glass dildo in their toy box. This is one of my personal favorites. It has the perfect curve and length to stimulate my G-spot, but its unique shape and design also make it perfect for anal stimulation as well.

www.pinkcherry.com/double-g-glass-stunner-in-pink

5. LIBERATOR BED BUCKLER TETHER AND CUFF RESTRAINT KIT

Another must-have for every toy box is an under-the-bed restraint kit. I'm a huge fan of Liberator because of the quality of products that they make. This set won't feel cheap or flimsy, and will last for years.

www.liberator.com/bed-buckler.html

6. LIBERATOR PLUSH SEDUCTION KIT

I would describe this set as plush but firm. The cuffs are extremely comfortable, but won't slip off, and the clips are so versatile that you can restrain your lover in any way that you can imagine. Again, it's from Liberator, so the quality of craftsmanship is excellent!

www.liberator.com/deluxe-plush-cuff-kit.html

7. DRAGONTAILZ LEATHER FLOGGER

Nothing beats the feel and smell of leather. This is a wonderful all-purpose flogger. From a relaxing massage to that magical sting on your skin, it's soft, yet sturdy enough to get the job done. You'll love this flogger for years to come.

www.liberator.com/dragontailz-balthazar-leather-flogger.html

8. ENJOY PURE PLUG 2.0

In addition to a glass toy, every toy box should have at least one metal toy. I prefer metal for anal play because it's near-indestructible and super easy to clean and disinfect. This one may be too big for beginners, but you'll easily work your way up to it.

www.liberator.com/njoy-pure-plug-2-0.html

9. LIBERATOR NJOY FUN WAND

The one toy I gave away and immediately regretted. . . . So, I got another one. Get one for yourself. You won't regret it.

www.liberator.com/njoy-fun-wand.html

10. PIPEDREAMS FETISH FANTASY SPINNING SEX SWING

Every couple needs a good sex swing, IMHO, and this one is just so versatile. If you haven't noticed, I like quality sex toys, and this is another one that you just can't go wrong with.

www.liberator.com/pipedream-fetish-fantasy-spinning-swing.html

ROB'S LIST

1. HOT OCTOPUSS—PULSE III DUO

The state-of-the-art vibrating male toy! The PULSE III Duo is designed to give men the pleasure that up to this point has been mainly focused on women. Vibration for men can be just as exciting as it is for women. However, the PULSE III Duo isn't just for the pleasure of men; this interesting new invention allows for both partners to enjoy the pleasure at the same time with a handheld remote that the woman controls to adjust the pleasure on the parts of her body, where she desires a little or a lot of extra sensation. As an added benefit, this toy has also been proven to help with erectile dysfunction in men as well.

www.hotoctopuss.com/pulse-iii/

2. LIBERATOR WEDGE & RAMP COMBO

If there is one item that every couple should have in their bedroom, it is the Liberator Wedge & Ramp Combo. This is one piece of furniture that comes in handy for almost all couples, allowing couples to experiment with different positions with ease. Individuals of all shapes and statures will find the Wedge & Ramp Combo success at helping to mix things up, and at adjusting angles of penetration in their sexual activity. Liberator makes the highest quality of bedroom furniture and accessories, and they also make sure the Wedge & Ramp combo are easy to clean. The Wedge and Ramp can also be used for stretching, yoga, or just relaxing, making it not only a help in your sex life, but in many other areas as well.

www.liberator.com/wedge-ramp-combo.html

3. FUN FACTORY—BOOTIE RING

For men, the Bootie Ring boasts the trifecta of pleasure. Helping you keep your erection firm and long-lasting with a silicone cock ring, the Bootie Ring also provides the excitement of anal stimulation and light prostate play, which creates a match made in heaven for both the man and his partner. The Bootie Ring adds the joy of perineum massage to the mix as well, making it a winner for the men who can't get enough pleasure.

us.funfactory.com/en/men-toys/bootie-ring/

4. FUN FACTORY—BI STRONIC FUSION

Bi Stronic Fusion combines the enjoyment of vibration, with the delightful rhythm of pulsation to help give women the best of both worlds. The strong pulsation of the Bi Stronic Fusion, coupled with the clit-vibrating appendage and the wings for stimulating the labia, is enough to send women over the top again and again. This is the ultimate power tool for women and men, so if you are always wanting more and more power in your tools, now you have one to share with your lady. Prepare for an abundance of sheet-gripping orgasms with this much power at your fingertips.

us.funfactory.com/en/pulsators/bi-stronic-fusion/

5. TENGA CUP SERIES

Tenga takes masturbation to a new level for men with their Cup Series. Now each experience can feel completely different. With a wide variety of inside textures, as well as different shapes, sizes, and friction levels, Tenga's Cup Series has a sensation for everyone. Tenga Cup Series also makes for a quick clean up afterwards. Women, you can join in the fun with the Tenga Cup Series, too, by giving your man a hand, and sharing in the pleasure of gliding the cups to pleasuring your man.

usstore.tenga-global.com/collections/one-time-disposables

6. IROHA TORI

The Iroha Tori takes comfort in sexual pleasure to another level. It's one of the softest intimate items you will ever have the pleasure of touching to your genitals. Combine that with a powerful motor and a variety of rhythmic patterns, and you have the touch of love with the Iroha Tori. It's soft enough to push into your pleasure centers, and with its unique design, creates pleasure in the form of artwork. The birdlike shape of this product also allows for it to get into any specific areas desired.

iroha-tenga.com/en/plus/

7. HONEY DUST BODY POWDER BY KAMA SUTRA

A wonderful body powder that makes you feel like a king or queen, Honey Dust by Kama Sutra brings the taste of sex to a place of utter delight. Lightly covering your skin with Honey Dust not only makes you feel fresh and exciting, it also makes you the most delicate of desserts for your lover. After applying Honey Dust, each kiss, smell, and lick of your partner will set both your lustful souls on fire.

kamasutra.com/collections/forplay/products/honey-dust-body-powder-6oz

8. CHAKRUBS

Chakrubs are the most spiritual of all the sex toys in this section, and maybe even in the world. Each Chakrub is crafted from natural crystals, which bring a sacredness to a couple's play time. Each Chakrub is handcrafted to allow the healing power to be shared during the most intimate of acts, allowing your body to connect and bond with the electromagnetic fields of our world and to the energy that encompasses our universe and beyond. Chakrubs might just be the most powerful sexual toy that you have ever owned.

www.chakrubs.com/the-original-chakrub-line/

9. ANEROS EUPHO TRIDENT

The Eupho Trident is a key to a prostate experience that men will find out of this world. With a slim body and soft, smooth curves, it makes even a beginner to the experience of prostate pleasure feel comfortable and at ease. The Eupho Trident can be used in solo play or can be experienced during the act of intercourse, giving double the pleasure. Enjoy the experience of longer and stronger orgasms with the Eupho Trident.

www.aneros.com/eupho-trident.html

10. INTIMATE EARTH—COLLECTION

For the truly earth-conscious lovers, the collection that Intimate Earth has to offer will make you into a love-crazed hippie. With products that are 100 percent vegan and that are never tested on animals, you can rest easy with the connection their products have with Mother Earth. However, you will also be pleasantly surprised at how amazing their products are. With their Oral Pleasure glides, Massage Oils, and Flavor Glide lubes, you will be treated with amazing tastes, feelings, and a well-oiled lovemaking experience. Don't forget about their line of Green Toy Cleaner to make your toys squeaky clean in the healthiest of ways, which is a pretty big deal.

www.intimate-earth.com/shop

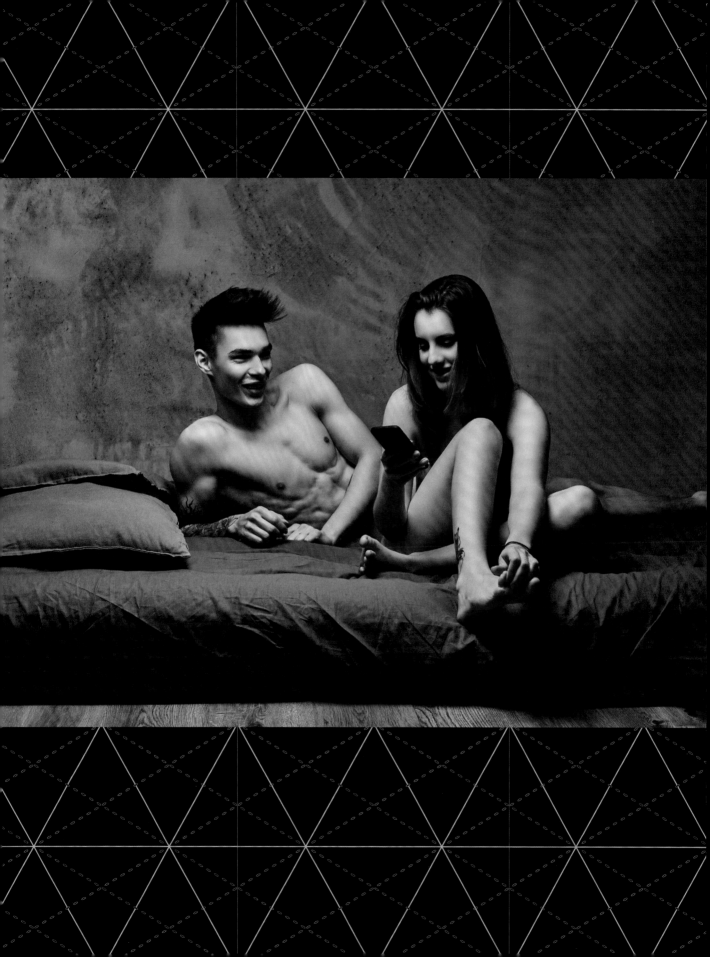

BEST SEX POSITIONS FOR OVERWEIGHT PEOPLE

While many of the positions in this book may be more challenging if you have some extra padding, there are still many options, and sex can still be creative and amazing. The secret is to focus on sex positions that get the job done, and still make you look and feel like a rock star.

Here are the ten best sex positions to try tonight if you've got some extra cushion for the pushin':

1. STANDING DOGGY

Try it leaning over a table or sofa arm. Both provide a sturdy and stable surface, and most of your weight is supported by your legs. It also allows her to easily spread her legs to the desired width to adjust for any height differences. If he has a bigger belly, she can bend over a little farther, so that his belly can ride over the top of her hips instead of getting in the way.

2. REVERSE COWGIRL

This is another great position if he has a bigger belly. Because she is leaning away from him, she moves down his legs to the point where his belly is no longer in the way. You can also add pillows or cushions under her knees to raise her body up, if needed, so that she can thrust more easily.

3. MISSIONARY

Missionary is super easy to modify, depending on what you need to work around. The trick is for him to support his weight on his forearms and knees. The more he bends his knees toward her hips, the more the bellies get out of the way. He can even sit up on his knees, if his arms start to get tired. Just keep adjusting the angle until you find what works.

4. MODIFIED BALLERINA

This standing sex position can easily be modified to make it more stable and easy to get into. Instead of standing straight up, she can lean onto her elbow using a counter-top or table. While she still needs to be flexible to get into this position, leaning on a solid surface opens all sorts of possibilities.

5. DEEP VICTORY

This is a great one because he can hold her legs straight up or wide open while standing at the edge of the bed or a table. To make this less stressful on her legs, you can add pillows or cushions under her legs and at the edge of her hips for support.

6. LAPTOP IN A SEX SWING

Laptop can be a tough position to get into if either of you are on the heavy side. By adding a sex swing, it takes all the pressure and weight off of you both. Just make sure to buy a quality swing and follow the installation instructions, so the swing is secure.

7. BUTTERFLY

The Butterfly is a simplified version of the bridge pose, and because she is supported and he is on his knees, the is a great position that anyone can do. Make sure to add a cushion under his knees for comfort.

8. DOGGY STYLE

This is one of the most popular sex positions for good reason. It feels great for both partners and can easily be modified to work around a bigger belly or voluptuous bottom. Try it with her on the bed, on hands and knees, with him standing behind her. She can adjust the height by bring her knees closer together or farther apart.

9. SPORK

The spork is a great position that allows both partners to rotate or slide around to find the best fit and angle of penetration. It's incredibly comfortable for both partners and can be used for vaginal or anal sex.

10. SCISSORS

Last but not least, the Scissors sex position opens things up and gets all those extra love handles out of the way. This is one of my favorites when she is pregnant because being on her side allows the baby to rest on the bed, so there is no pressure on mom's back!

Getting in the Flow

(How to Transition Through Multiple Positions)

Within the pages of this book, you have seen many amazing sexual positions, and you can use each and every one to satisfaction during your intimate experience. However, there is an energy to our sex that loves to flow and move around our bodies, taking us to places that we have never been. Think about a massage: if you only get your shoulders worked, then afterwards your shoulders feel great, but an entire body massage makes your entire body feel amazing. With that in mind, we want to challenge you to get in the flow of sex by learning how certain positions can work together, so you can move from one to the other without stopping the excitement and passion from flowing.

Now, when we are talking about switching positions, we want you to break out of each section. By that, we mean that we don't want you to switch from one of the missionary positions to the next missionary position. We want you to think outside the sexual box. Get out of the mindset of normal. For example, many couples might enjoy oral sex, but they usually will have it, and then go to the standard missionary position, and that is fine. But, if you want to use the flow of sex to really create great things, then start switching things up. Based on the example above, who says you can't switch from the missionary position back to having oral sex? Nobody, and let me tell you, it is highly arousing.

When you switch positions during the flow of sex, you do more than just change positions. You change the angle of penetration, so that both partners get a different feel on their genitals. They also allow you to touch and experience your partner's other parts, such as their breasts, butt, and face, in many different ways.

Changing positions can also change the speed of sex, since one position might allow you to be moving and thrusting fast, and the next one might force you to go a little slower and thrust a little deeper, again creating many different sensations during the entire sexual act. By switching positions in an outside-the-box manner, you can roll many sensations into one night of sex.

Just remember—this is super important for the guys—you don't have to climax or have an orgasm in each position. While several of the women reading this might be able to do that, not very many men can. So, guys, don't think about switching positions as a challenge to see how many times you can ejaculate in an evening, because that number will be low for many of you. Think of it as a way of creating a long-lasting sexual experience of epic status. This is also great to help give your female partner more time than ever to enjoy the flow.

Now, spontaneous movement from one position to another would be amazingly awesome. You also don't want to be lying in bed trying to figure out what position you should try next. Idle time in bed isn't usually productive, especially once the festivities have started; remember, there is a flow to all this. We don't want minutes between sexual positions, with time for heart rates to return to normal, or having to re-heat the oven on those partners who take a while to heat up. My advice is to have a plan and not leave this to chance. Sit down as part of your foreplay, and go through this book and pick some positions you want to try during the evening.

We are going to give you some examples of position flow to help you get started. From that point, you can keep going back to these or you can start creating your own.

THE DELIGHTFUL–BULLDOG–CLIMBING THE FLAGPOLE FLOW. Begin with your partner using the Delight missionary position. This position has lots of eye contact and allows for lots of kissing and touching. At this point, the female partner can turn around, climb up a little on the bed, and the man can come up from behind and get into the Bulldog-Rear-Entry Position. To finish off this trifecta, the woman would just turn over to her side and raise one leg into the air, inviting her partner to enter her in the Climbing-the-Flagpole, Deep-Penetration Position. This flow allows for a building of pleasure that should result in a climatic end.

THE ORAL PRESENTATION FLOW. If you both love oral sex, this is the flow for the both of you. Start out in the Reverse-69 position, allowing both partners to get excited and super juicy for this flow. The next move is for the female to raise up and slip into the Reverse Face Straddle from the "Oral Sex Positions for Her" section. Then, after the woman is pleasured and satisfied, she should roll off her partner and allow him to move his genitals up to her face, getting into the Face Straddle for Him from the "Oral Sex Positions for Men." In this flow, you can pleasure each other to climax orally, or you can add another position to the end, to allow you both the opportunity to climax or orgasm.

THE SEA LIFE SEXY FLOW. This Sea Life-themed flow has some great sensations to it; you might want to even call them waves of pleasure. Let's begin by getting into the Turtle Position from the "Rear Entry" section of the book. This is a nice warm up to this sexual flow, as it is a slow build to arousal. Next, let's turn up the heat a little by moving to the Crab Position from the "Woman on Top" section. This position is very erotic, as it allows both partners to see the pleasure on each other's face, yet keeps their faces a distance apart so they can enjoy watching the action. We move on from the woman-dominant position of the Crab to the male dominant position of the Viennese Oyster from the "Deep-Penetration" sex positions section. This position will really turn your male partner on and it's a great one to help him reach climax. So, ladies, you might focus on your climax during the Crab Position. After this position, you might want to go check out the local seafood restaurant just for fun.

HOW THE WEST WAS WON FLOW. In this flow, you might want to dust off your boots and maybe wear your spurs if you like, because we are going to create our own little rodeo. I just hope it last longer than eight seconds for you. Saddle up ladies, you're first as we move into the Cowgirl Position, and allow the ladies to buck and rock their way to pleasure in this Lady-on-Top position. Next, guys, it's time for you to grab the reins and hightail it into the Cowboy Position from the "Missionary Position" section. Finally, it is time for a little wilder ride as we move to the Reverse Jockey Position from the "Rear-Entry" Position section. Together the two of you will tame the West and defiantly knock the dust off your saddles. Another playful way to add excitement to this flow is to add a little roping and tying up of your partner.

THE SPIRITUAL JOURNEY SEXUAL FLOW. Our Sexual Experiences are always a journey; they allow us to experience things we don't in our day to day life. This flow takes some of the positions from the book that closely resemble yoga poses and makes them into a sexual flow of out-of-this-world pleasure. First, let's start by getting into the Lotus Position from the "Sitting Sexual Positions" sections. These positions allow both partners to connect in a very deep spiritual manner and is great for the start of this flow. Next, let's move to the Coital Alignment Technique, which can be a very spiritual position, especially for the women out there. Finally, we move to the Yoga-Master Position from the "Rear-Entry" section, which is a very difficult position, but one that can connect a couple in amazing ways.

OK, you now have five different Sexual Flows to use in your sexual practices. This is by no means the end of the list. We encourage you to make up your own flows and be creative. We have used three positions in all our flows, but you can do many more if you like. The beautiful part about the flow of sexual energy is that it can take you to many fabulous places, allowing couples to experience highs that they never thought they would be able to achieve. There is something super exciting about being naked with your partner and doing this dance of passion together.

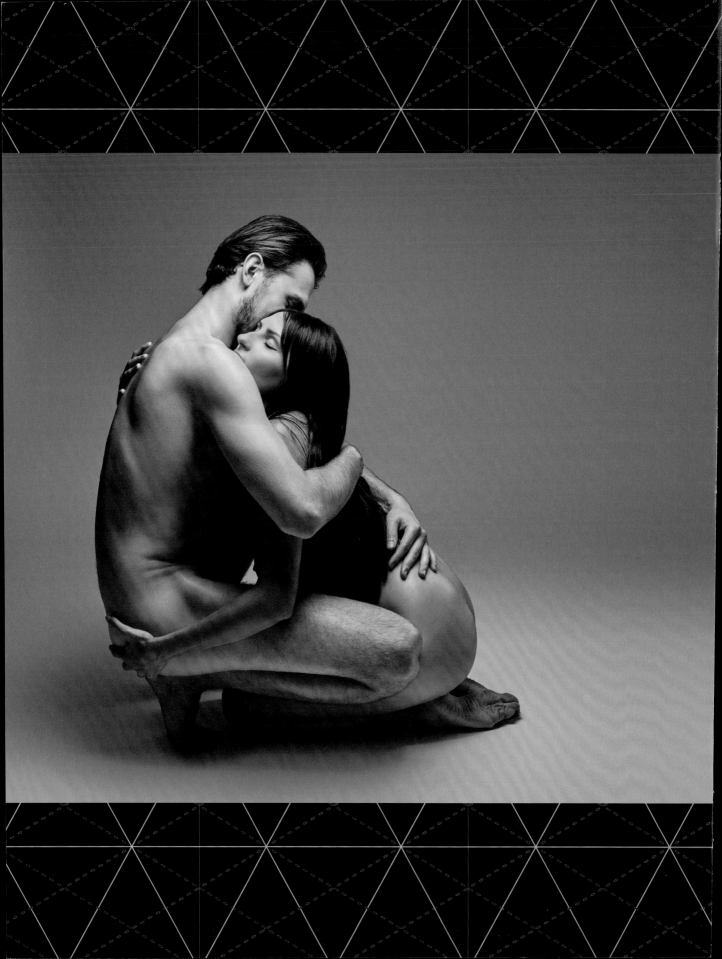

ABOUT THE AUTHORS

JENNIFER BARITCHI is the founder and senior editor of LoveAndSex-Answers.com, which has been referred to as "The Best & Most Popular Dating, Love, and Sex Advice Column on the Internet Today . . ." She has been a full-time author and blogger since 2006 and has helped millions of people enjoy amazing sex and more fulfilling relationships.

Other books by Jennifer Baritchi:
The Little Black Book of Sex Positions
1001 Best Places to Have Sex in America
The Best Sex of Your Life
Follow Jennifer on Amazon:
www.amazon.com/Jennifer-Baritchi/e/B003K1GS02/

ROB ALEX, PhD, has been helping couples have amazing relationships since 2008, when he started a blog called "The Couples Spot." As his passion for helping people have more fulfilling relationships and sex lives grew, he created Sexy Challenges in 2009. With over half a million downloads of Sexy Challenges on iTunes and Amazon, he continues to change the landscape of sex and relationships. With a PhD. in Metaphysical Sciences, Rob gives individuals and couples the chance to get outside the box within intimacy.

Rob has also been the host of two top-ten podcasts on iTunes, instructs classes, and is known as one of the worst karaoke singers of all time. His Mission Date Night Adventures, which create effortless memorable date nights for couples, was considered for the show *Shark Tank*. With his passion for passion, Rob is helping to create amazing sexual energy all around the world. You can find Rob's Sexy Challenges and other books on Amazon and iTunes, and you can keep up with his crazy busy life at sexychallenges.com

Other Books by Rob Alex, PhD
The Top 100 Intimate Items for Lovers—FREE Book
Sexy Challenges—Sacred and Sensual Experiences for lovers
Sexy Challenges 33 Adventures : Create Powerful Energy with Passion, Purpose and Love
Speaking Kind Words
The Full Moon Approaches: Merging Moon Energy, Earth Energy & Sexual Energy
Motivating Yourself the Sexy Way
Keep up with Sexy Challenges at sexychallenges.com
Follow Rob on Amazon:
www.amazon.com/Rob-Alex-Ph.D./e/B00OPTQKT2/